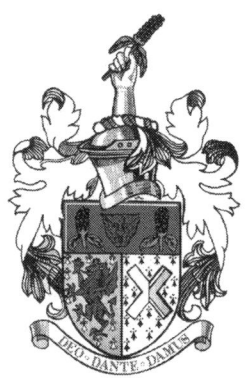

Spinal Disorders for Beginners
The Oswestry Spine Primer

Stephen Eisenstein

PhD FRCS

Institute of Orthopaedics (Oswestry) Publishing Group
Institute of Orthopaedics
The Robert Jones and Agnes Hunt
Orthopaedic Hospital Oswestry
Shropshire SY10 7AG

2012

First published in 2012 by
Institute of Orthopaedics (Oswestry) Publishing Group,
Institute of Orthopaedics,
The Robert Jones and Agnes Hunt Orthopaedic Hospital,
Oswestry, Shropshire SY10 7AG

Copyright Stephen Eisenstein 2012 ©
Images permission granted to Institute of Orthopaedics publishing group

All rights reserved. No part of this publication may be reproduced, stored in a retrieval system, or transmitted, in any form, or by any means, electronic, mechanical, photo copying, recording or otherwise, without the prior permission of the publisher and copyright holder.

British Library Cataloguing in Publication data
A catalogue record for this book is available from the British Library.

ISBN-13: 978-1481120432

DEDICATION

Louis Solomon

George Dommisse

Brian O'Connor

John O'Brien

Helen Rooney

INTRODUCTION

This pocket book is intended to appeal to all practitioners in Primary Care because of a perceived deficiency of information on spinal disorders stripped of the customary mystique. The vocabulary and the practise of spinal disorders, especially in the management of back pain, remain esoteric subjects for many doctors not specialised in this area. The inherent difficulty in providing patients with a diagnosis for the pains so frequently and vociferously complained of, together with the customary absence of identifiable pathology, render this discipline the last great cause for dismay in our colleagues everywhere but particularly in primary care. The possibility of missing the diagnosis of a rare instance of serious and potentially crippling spinal illness adds fear and apprehension to the existing frustration. This situation is probably not much alleviated by the fact of minimal provision for musculoskeletal subjects in undergraduate education.

Although some excellent pamphlets are now available to instruct doctors in the assessment and management of back pain, there is no publication of this kind covering all spinal disorders. There are indeed recent titles advertised as "primers" simply because all the voluminous information is contained in one closely printed bulky volume.

- **The purpose of this primer is to guide the reader through the issues and the esoteric terminology** relevant to all the spinal disorders, in a simple and direct manner, so that readers can make the subject their own after brief study. Demystification is the theme.
- **Opinions are frequent,** based on personal experience not necessarily supported by published research, and in all instances attributable to the author.
- **The major headings are presented in alphabetical order** for ease of access. To this end there is also a glossary, and sections on acronyms, eponyms, and jargon.

- **The booklet is much illustrated**, especially with the radiographic and scan images which constitute the single chief diagnostic method in spinal disorders. Primary care doctors in Britain have little opportunity to become acquainted with the finer points of radiological diagnosis: they may relish the opportunity to acquire some expertise with little additional effort. Indeed, the NICE (National Institute for Clinical Excellence) guidelines for the "Early Management of persistent non-specific Low back Pain" (May 2009) discourage all X-rays at primary care level, while promoting MRI on suspicion, at £500 plus per spinal region.
  The guidelines offer little advance on the algorithm as shown on page 23.
- **Where appropriate, algorithms are offered**, provided they can be kept very simple. Some algorithms available in some major textbooks are rendered entirely pointless by their complexity.
- **The section on eponyms** is provided for diversion and education beyond the merely utilitarian.
- **Bold typeface** within the text is used to indicate words explained more fully in the GLOSSARY, or under ACRONYMS, or under EPONYMS.
- **References** to the published literature are few: this is not a text book, and further reading is so easily accessible via the internet.
- **Although the author is a spinal surgeon, contributors include a senior General Practitioner with a special interest in spinal disorders, an Allied Health Professional spinal surgical practitioner, and a medical student**. These contributors have been chosen to assist the author to retain focus and direction appropriate to the purposes of this publication.

- **It remains the hope of the author that this publication will find some use also among surgical trainees, senior medical students, and members of the lay public.**

ACKNOWLEDGMENTS

MAJOR CONTRIBUTORS
VICTOR CASSAR-PULLICINO, Consultant Radiologist, The Robert Jones and Agnes Hunt Orthopaedic Hospital, Oswestry.
JAYESH TRIVEDI, Consultant Spine Surgeon and Director, Department for Spinal Disorders, The Robert Jones and Agnes Hunt Orthopaedic Hospital, Oswestry.
DAVID CAMPBELL, General Practitioner with special interest in Spinal Disorders, Oswestry.
WAGIH S EL MASRY, Director, Midland Centre for Spinal Cord Injury, The Robert Jones and Agnes Hunt Orthopaedic Hospital, Oswestry.
ALUN JONES and **ANDREW BIGGS**, Medical Illustrators, The Robert Jones and Agnes Hunt Orthopaedic Hospital, Oswestry.

CONTRIBUTORS
Caroline Lesley Evans, Surgical Assistant and Superintendent Physiotherapist, Lead Practitioner in Functional Restoration Programme.
David Jaffray, Consultant Spine Surgeon.
Birender Balain, Consultant Spine Surgeon.
Iain McCall Consultant radiologist.
Marie Carter and colleagues, Librarians, Orthopaedic Institute, The Robert Jones and Agnes Hunt Orthopaedic Hospital, Oswestry.
John Kirkup, Curator, Royal College of Surgeons Hunterian Museum, London.
James Edmonson, Curator, Dittrick Museum, Case Western Reserve University, Cleveland, USA.
Eva Eisenstein, Research Librarian, Evanston Northwestern Healthcare Research Institute, Illinois, USA.
Neil Eisenstein, Year 6 medical student, Jesus College, Oxford.

PUBLICATIONS
Stedman's Medical Dictionary 27th Edition 2000, Lippincott Williams & Wilkins, Philadelphia.
Gray's Anatomy 35th Ed. Warwick R, Williams P Eds. 1973. Longmans. Edinburgh.
Tumors of the Spine Eds. Sundaresan N, Schmidek H, Schiller A, Rosenthal D. 1990 W.B.Saunders Company, Philadelphia.
Myofascial Pain and Dysfunction. Travell J.G. Simons D.G. Baltimore, Williams & Wilkins. 1983.

CONTENTS

	Page
Introduction.	4
Acknowledgements.	6
Contents.	7
Acronyms.	9
Anatomy and Physiology.	11
Ankylosing Spondylitis.	17
Arthritis.	21
Back Pain/Lower limb complex.	23
Back Pain - General.	25
Back Pain - High.	29
Back Pain - Low.	31
Cancer.	36
Cauda Equina Syndrome.	36
Coccyx and Coccydynia.	38
Complementary Therapies.	39
Complications.	40
Consent.	46
Disability, Impairment, Incapacity and Handicap.	48
Disc.	50
Discitis.	56
Embryology.	60
Emergencies.	65
Epidural Abscess.	66
Eponyms.	68
Examination.	78
Failed Lumbar Surgery Algorithm for Management.	84
Functional Restoration.	85
Glossary.	87
History.	93
Imaging.	96
Infection.	102
Imflammatory Arthritis.	102
Jargon and Misnomers.	104
Kyphosis.	106
Lordosis.	107
MRI Vertbral Marrow Signal Change.	108
Muscle Power.	109

	Page
Neck and Upper Limb Pain.	110
Non Spinal Backpain and Sciatica.	112
Osteomyelitis.	114
Osteoporosis	117
Oswestry Disability Index (ODI).	119
Paralysis and Spinal Cord injury	123
Physiotherapy.	123
Pseudarthrosis.	124
Posture.	125
Sciatica.	126
Scoliosis.	129
Spina Bifida.	144
Spondylitis.	146
Spondylolisthesis.	149
Spondylolysis.	152
Spondylosis.	156
Stenosis.	157
Surgery.	161
Surgery Stabilisation.	167
Trauma.	172
Tumour - Primary.	181
Tumour - Metastasis.	183
Whiplash.	190
Wound Infection.	192
X-Rays.	193
Zoster.	193

ACRONYMS

Are shortcuts in speaking and writing whereby the names of diseases, tests, institutions, and concepts are reduced to their first letter abbreviations. The unintended side effect is an element of secrecy, and knowledge available only to the initiated.

ADL	Activities of Daily Living.
AIDS	Acquired Immune Deficiency Syndrome.
ALIF	Anterior Lumbar Interbody Fusion.
ASIA	American Spinal Injury Association. Applies generally to a score for severity of spinal cord injury, but probably of no greater usefulness than the Frankel grading.
BMD	Bone Mineral Density.
BMI	Body Mass Index: weight (kg) divided by height squared (metres^2). N adults = 18.5-24.9.
BMP	Bone Morphogenic Protein.
BNF	British National Formulary (pharmaceuticals).
COAD	Chronic Obstructive Airways Disease.
CPK	Creatine Phosphokinase.
CRP	C-Reactive Protein.
CSF	Cerebrospinal Fluid.
CT	Computerised Tomography.
DEXA	Dual Energy X-ray Absorptiometry.
DISH	Diffuse Idiopathic Skeletal Hyperostosis/Forestier's Disease.
DLA	Disability Living Allowance.
DVT	Deep Vein Thrombosis.
DWP	Department of Work and Pensions.
ESR	Erythrocyte Sedimentation Rate.
FBC	Full Blood Count.
FDA	Federal Drug Administration (USA.)
FRP	Functional Restoration Programme.
IVP	Intravenous Pyelogram.
MIMS	Monthly Index of Medical Specialties (pharmaceuticals).
MRC	Medical Research Council muscle power grading: (see under MUSCLE POWER.)
MRI	Magnetic Resonance Imaging.
MRSA	Methicillin Resistant Staphylococcus Aureus.
HLA B27	Human Lymphocyte Antigen. Typical serum finding in ankylosing spondylitis.
LFT	Liver Function Test.
NICE	National Institute for Clinical Exellence.
OPLL	Ossification Posterior Longitudinal Ligament, usually cervical spine, Japanese.

PCA	Patient Controlled Analgesia.
PE	Pulmonary Embolus.
PEEK	Phenyl Ether Ether Ketone. Material for interbody cages.
PET	Positron Emission Tomography.
PICC	Peripherally Inserted Central (venous) Catheter.
PLIF	Posterior Lumbar Interbody Fusion.
	Developed by Ralph B Cloward, neurosurgeon.
RTA	Road Traffic Accident.
U&E	Urea and Electrolytes.
WHO	World Health Organisation.

ANATOMY & PHYSIOLOGY

The human spine represents a marvel of evolutionary development for multiple functions. The spine must protect its vital neural contents as best possible while allowing strenuous weight bearing and movement through a wide range of postures and contortions. It must continue strong and flexible for what has become double the designed life of the four decades of early man. It is not surprising therefore if there are some difficulties to be found along the way in the form of pain, deformity, and disintegration in varying proportions for many individuals. These difficulties constitute the spinal disorders to which this booklet is directed.

The spine consists of roughly 24 stacked bony rings (vertebrae) connected by ligaments. There are three groups of vertebrae, according to geographical location, going from top to bottom (proximal to distal): 7 cervical; 12 thoracic; 5 lumbar. The number may vary between individuals by one or two. These variations are to be found at the zones of transition between the three groups.

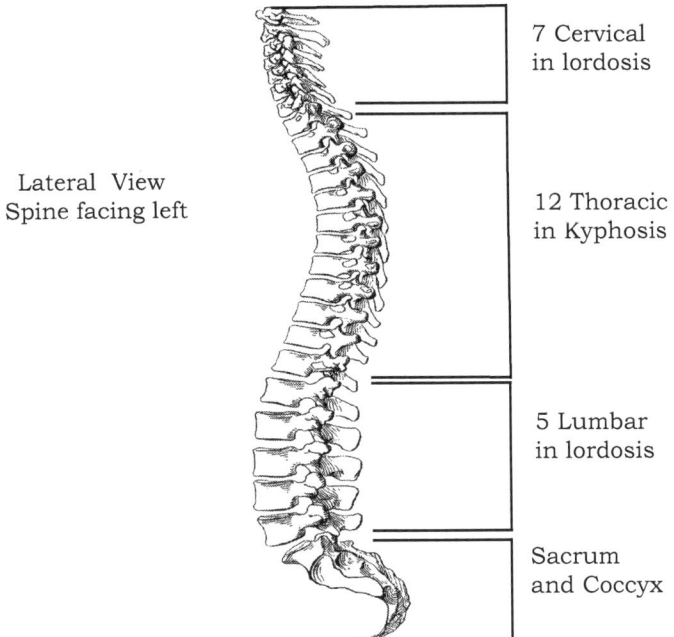

Lateral View
Spine facing left

7 Cervical
in lordosis

12 Thoracic
in Kyphosis

5 Lumbar
in lordosis

Sacrum
and Coccyx

Anatomy & Physiology

Transitional variation is anatomically interesting but seldom of clinical significance, even at the lumbosacral junction, despite fond belief to the contrary. When a fifth lumbar vertebra is attached to the sacrum by a sacrotransverse bar or joint, that is called sacralisation. Similarly, when a first sacral segment is partially separated from the sacrum, that is called lumbarisation. The frequency of lumbosacral transitional variation averages 10% across Caucasoid and Negroid populations and both genders (Eisenstein SM. J Bone Joint Surg 1977, 59-B:173-80).

The bony rings all have the same basic design, to provide stability against gravity and strain, and allow passage of the spinal cord and cauda equina. Vertebrae are thickened in front (anteriorly) to form a block of bone (body), and carry a posterior projection (spinous process) for the attachment of ligaments and muscles. Lateral projections from most of the rings are the transverse processes, serving a similar purpose. At the root of the transverse processes are platforms with smooth cartilage covering their surfaces ("facets" reminiscent of polished gemstones). Articulating surfaces of adjacent vertebrae, enclosed by a fibrous capsule, make a facet joint. Again, from the base of the transverse processes are bars of bone going forwards (pedicles) to join up to the bodies, and blades of bone going backwards (laminae) making an arch peaking at the base of the spinous process. A narrow waist in the lamina is pars interarticularis (the part between the facet joints), frequently fractured in childhood and causing back pain in later life. The pedicles and the laminae make up the bony posterior boundaries of the spinal canal.

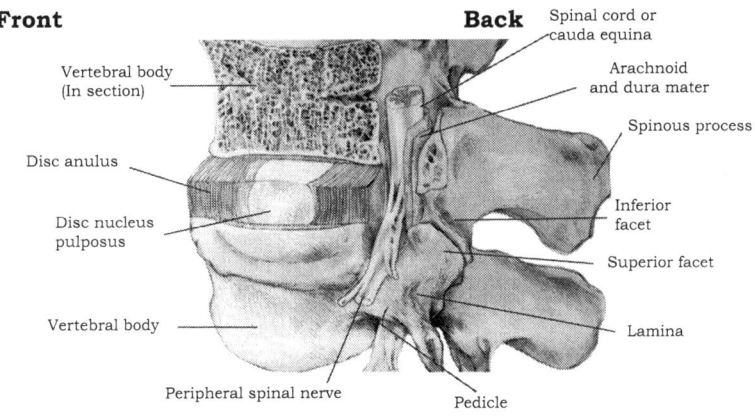

Anatomy & Physiology

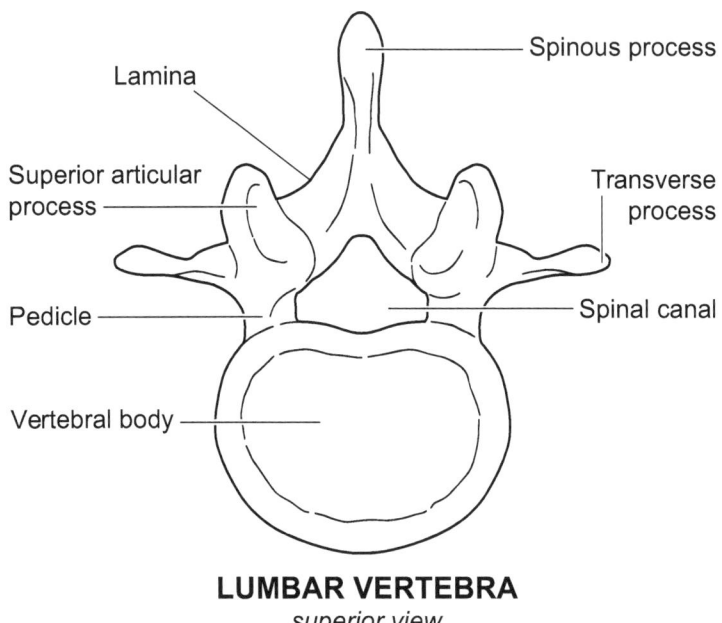

LUMBAR VERTEBRA
superior view

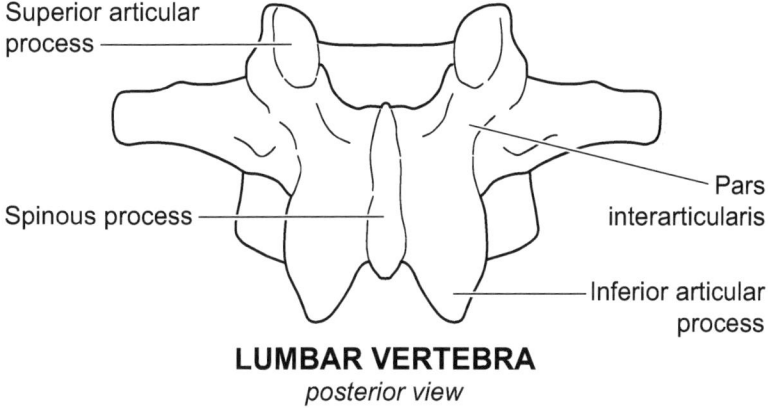

LUMBAR VERTEBRA
posterior view

The vertebral bodies are connected by a highly organised ligamentous ring (anulus) of alternating layers of obliquely aligned fibres, enclosing in turn a tough hydrophilic collagen gel (nucleus), together named the intervertebral disc. Discs increase in height and cross-sectional area from top to bottom, as one might expect, except that the last disc (L5S1) is slightly smaller again. This makes the L4/5 disc the largest avascular structure in the human body. Water constitutes 90% of the bulk of the normal disc and acts as a kind of hydraulic fluid in the spine. The water is drawn in powerfully by hydrophilic proteoglycans in the nucleus of the disc. It is likely that most back pain of middle age and beyond begins with some loss of this water. The longitudinal ligaments, anterior and posterior, run the length of the spine adherent to anterior and posterior surfaces of the bodies and discs.

This general anatomical configuration is altered at the top end of the cervical spine, where C1 has surrendered its body to be welded on top of the existing body of C2. This upright projection acts as a pivot (odontoid) peg inside the ring of C1, and is held there by ligaments. This arrangement allows the head with C1 (the atlas), to rotate left/right on C2 (the axis) to at least half the range allowed by the whole cervical spine. The lateral limits of the C1 ring (atlas) carry upward facing facets which articulate with corresponding occipital facets of the skull, to allow flexion/extension of the head.

Normal stance in lateral projection reveals forward and backward curves from top to bottom of the spine, but still allowing the head to balance on the sacrum, more or less. These curves are **lordosis** in the cervical and lumbar spine, **kyphosis** in the thoracic spine. The accepted upper limit of the kyphosis (backward curve) in the thoracic spine is $40°$.

The thoracic vertebrae also have small modifications from the general pattern, if only to remind us that the head and neck of the ribs articulate with the body and transverse process respectively, at small articular surfaces. The unsightly rib hump of scoliosis is the result of these attachments forcing up the ribs on one side when the spine develops a curvature. The ribs attach to the sternum (breast bone) anteriorly, so that the rib cage does indeed provide a significant splinting protection for the thoracic spine, against injury.

Osteology reminds us that bony prominences invariably serve the purpose of ligamentous attachment. The spinous processes give attachment to the interspinous and supraspinous ligaments, and thereby (in the lumbar spine) directly to the lumbar fascia and the whole abdominal control of trunk stability. It is logical therefore, where possible, to preserve the posterior midline during posterior surgery.

The sacrum serves not only as the central wedge of the pelvis but also as the continuation of the spinal anatomy. It consists of approximately five fused bony segments, still holed sufficiently to allow the passage of segmental nerves serving the sciatic nerve and pelvic viscera. The sacrum gives some purchase for the foundation of the spine, but the iliac crests provide a great deal more, in the form of purchase for the lumbar fascia and iliolumbar ligaments. The sacroiliac joints are a favourite blameworthy source of pain, but the massive ligamentous attachments to the iliac crests are probably a much greater source of pain through strain injuries: <u>"tennis elbow" of the spine, in the "Bermuda Triangle" of lumbosacral pain.</u>

The spine ends in the coccyx, a small spur of miniature vertebrae, largely redundant and representing the developmental remnant of a tail. The coccygeal segments may be all fused together like the sacrum, but may continue as up to four separate pieces. The fact remains that the pelvic floor attaches to the sides of the coccyx. It is likely that many instances of disabling pain in the coccyx (coccydynia) originate in strain injuries of the pelvic floor such as in pregnancy and labour. The coccyx articulates with the end of the sacrum by a mixed anatomy of disc and synovial joints, a further source of coccydynia, especially after direct injury. This articulation can show the coccyx taking up some strange positions on x-ray, so frequently that none of them can be considered inherently abnormal or pathological. (See also p.38).

ANKYLOSING SPONDYLITIS (AS)

1. Inflammatory disease of spine and pelvic sacro-iliac joints, leading ultimately to spontaneous bony fusion (ankylosis).
2. Genetically predisposed, in Caucasoids, associated with presence of HLA B27 antigen.
3. Onset 15 – 25 years, spontaneous; male/female ratio approx 3:1.
4. Regarded as one of the rheumatoid diseases. Also known as rheumatoid spondylitis (too easily confused with the spondylitis of rheumatoid arthritis).
5. Is a generalised musculoskeletal and joint disease, a frequently forgotten aspect. Other joints possibly involved in inflammatory destruction are hips, knees and shoulders.
6. Clinical presentation, early, is generalised "aches and pains" and stiffness, especially spinal. Athletes may complain of unexplained breathlessness.
7. Clinical presentation, late, is characteristic thoracic **kyphosis** deformity with loss of forward gaze, and dramatic stiffness. Pain may be less than in early stage AS, but severe pain may indicate a persistent pseudarthrosis within an ankylosed segment. Hip joint stiffness may contribute to generalised kyphosis.

Diagnosis
- Clinical suspicion: young adult with too much unexplained back pain.
- Sacro-iliac joints may be sensitive to direct pressure, or painful when using hip joint stresses. **Schober's** test for lumbar spine stiffness is positive (see EPONYMS). Chest excursion maximum is less than 5 centimetres in adult, measured by tape just below nipples/breasts.
Plain x-ray pelvis shows unmistakable signs of sacroiliitis (sclerosis and lysis), or complete ankylosis before any change seen in spine itself.

Ankylosing Spondylitis

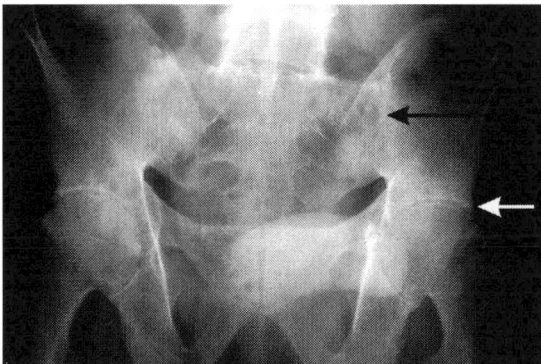

Obliterated ankylosed sacro-iliac joint

Imflammatory hip arthritis of AS.

- IF SYMPTOMS HAVE BEEN PRESENT FOR 18 MONTHS, SACRO-ILIITIS WILL BE VISIBLE IF THE DIAGNOSIS IS ANKYLOSING SPONDYLITIS. Early sign in the spine is the exaggeratedly square appearance of vertebral bodies ("**Romanus** lesion") owing to AS **enthesitis.**
- Plain x-ray spine in later stages: unmistakeable symmetrical ankylosis across intervertebral discs at their anular margins ("bamboo spine"); obliteration of facet joint spaces; thoracic kyphosis; cervical kyphosis; loss of lumbar lordosis.

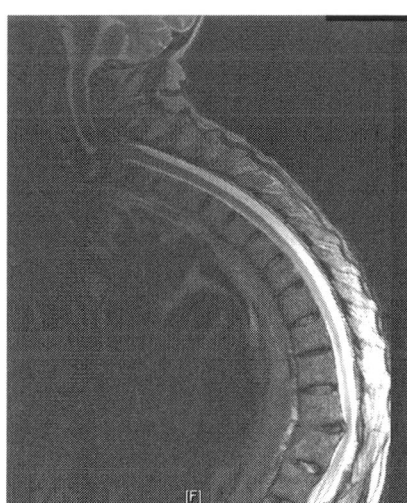

Rigid thoracic kyphosis with square vertebral bodies

18

Ankylosing Spondylitis

- Positive HLA B27 serology is confirmatory but not necessary for diagnosis. ESR raised in acute phases. Rheumatoid Factor negative.

Differential Diagnosis
- Low back strain: should resolve spontaneously within weeks.
- Spondylolysis/Spondylolisthesis.
- Ankylosing Hyperostosis/DISH/**Forestier's** Disease: large asymmetrical **syndesmophytes** discovered incidentally; very little pain.
- Seronegative spondylarthropathies: Reiter's; Crohn's; Behcet's syndrome; Psoriatic arthropathy; Ulcerative colitis.

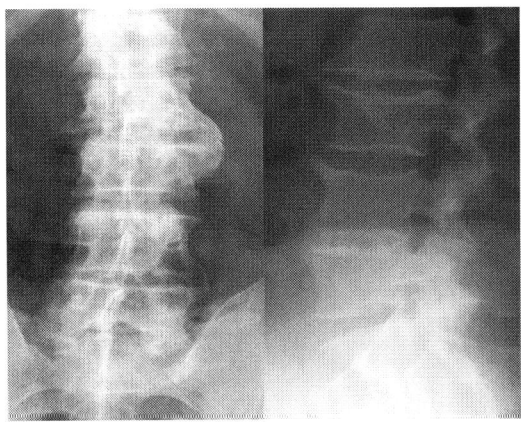

Ankylosing Hyperostosis

Treatment
- Intensive exercise regimen in early stages, emphasising spinal extension.
- Standard analgesics and anti-inflammatory medications for pain.
- Surgery: extension osteotomy and fusion at midlumbar spine (and/or cervicothoracic junction) when forward gaze lost to the point of significant disability High complication rate from paralysis, loss of fixation in accompanying osteoporosis, acute injury to stretched aorta. Surgery contra-indicated in presence of aortic calcification.

Ankylosing Spondylitis

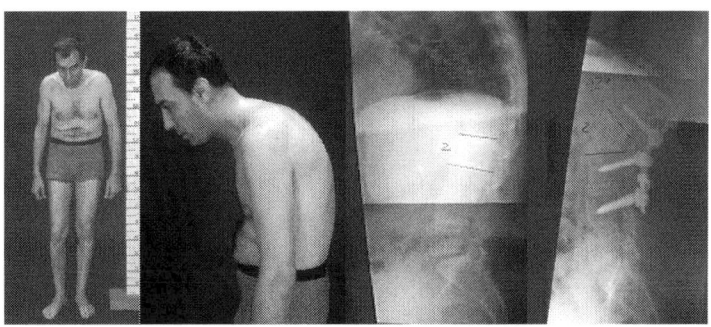

Pre - op   Lumbar Closing Wedge Osteotomy

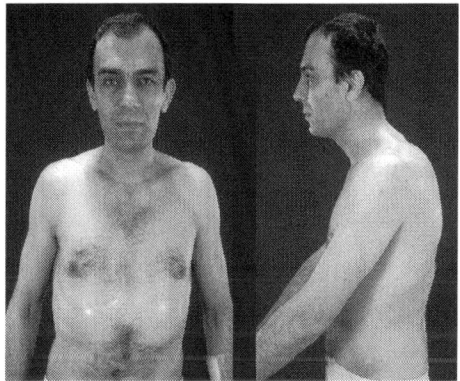

Post - op

- Surgery consists of closing wedge osteotomy, rather than previous **Smith-Petersen** opening wedge. Chosen vertebral body eg L3 is entered posteriorly via pedicles and emptied of bone by curette, followed by excision of medial walls of pedicles, crushing of posterior wall of vertebral body, forced extension at that site and fixation in corrected position.
- Surgical fusion operation (cruel irony) may be required for painful persistent spontaneous pseudarthrosis.
- Successful surgery produces very grateful patients.

ARTHRITIS

[see also SPONDYLOSIS, SPONDYLITIS, and INFLAMMATORY ARTHRITIS]

- This is the diagnosis most dreaded by the lay public, after cancer. This fear represents a cultural phenomenon, reinforced by unjustified warnings of a "crumbling spine" and a wheelchair existence unless the greatest care is taken.
- These inappropriate warnings are sometimes issued by doctors, perhaps with the best intentions, but thereby creating a whole new area of disability unnecessarily.
- Very rarely, a patient suffering widespread inflammatory (especially rheumatoid) arthritis may indeed achieve greater mobility in a wheelchair.
- Too often, doctors read a radiologist's report of "O/A spine" to the patient, honestly believing that they are providing the patient with the reassurance that there is no evidence of cancer.
- In the vast majority of cases, the "arthritis" referred to is nothing more than SPONDYLOSIS ie "wear-and-tear", the passage of time, and a bit of bad luck (because many people with spondylosis have little or no pain from it).

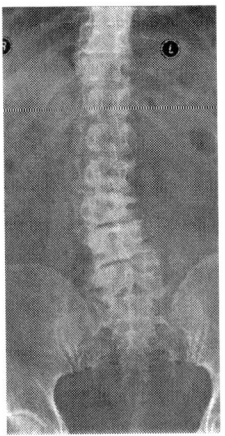 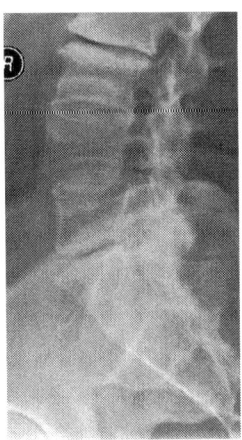

Plain X-ray lumbar spine.
AP and Lateral: spondylosis in elderly female.

Arthritis

- The back pain and neck pain that can be associated with SPONDYLOSIS may not be curable but usually can be *managed* to the point where it no longer constitutes a disability.
- The management of this spinal pain begins with the assurance that there is no detectable *disease* in the spine (even if plain x-rays and **MRI** are required to serve this purpose).
- Management continues with a variable combination of mild manipulative therapies (provided by any who have the skills, including physiotherapists, chiropractors, and osteopaths); analgesic medication; and infiltration of common trigger points with steroid and local anaesthetic.
- Surgery in the form of spinal fusion is available for a certain level of desperation experienced by the patient when all above has failed and disability of a high order rules all of daily life (see SURGERY – STABILISATION).

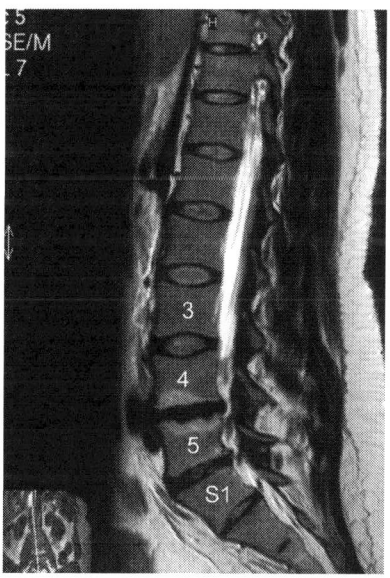

Sagittal MRI: spondylosis L4/5 L5/S1

BACK/LOWER LIMB PAIN COMPLEX
PRIMARY CARE ALGORITHM

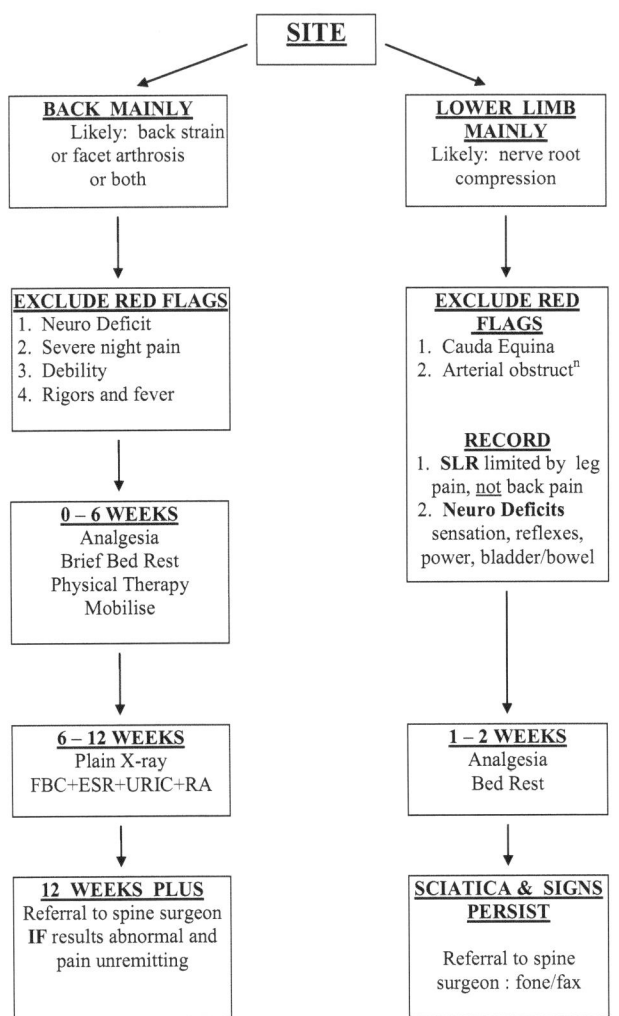

© *Stephen Eisenstein*
Eisenstein S. Low back pain algorithm for primary care. J. Bone Joint Surg 1998, 80B Suppl 2, 150.

Back / Lower limb pain complex

The algorithm is self-explanatory but some short notes are in order:-

- The **first step** is to seek clarity from the patient, through careful questioning, as to whether the symptoms are maximal in the **low back** area or in the **lower limb**. If the latter, we may be dealing with a nerve root compression which will need a diagnostic and therapeutic approach rather different from that which would apply to common low back pain.

- The **second step** requires us to deal with **"red flags"** ie those symptoms and signs which suggest some uncommon but far more serious disease eg CANCER, INFECTION, CAUDA EQUINA syndrome, and arterial obstructive disease.

- Ask about weight loss, loss of appetite, night pain, rigors, sweats, perineal and peri-anal sensation, bladder and bowel control, weakness in lower limbs.

- Assess peripheral lower limb pulses in every patient, as a matter of habit.

- Diagnostic methods are increased in stages, depending on the duration and severity of the symptoms, and always with the "red flag" symptoms and signs in mind.

- Referral to spine surgeon should be more urgent in suspected nerve root compression than for common low back pain, for the simple reason that the pain of nerve root compression is frequently unendurable.

- Referral should include a basic set of plain x-rays of lumbar spine and pelvis, to enable the surgeon to exclude some obvious explanatory pathology eg infiltrative disease, spondylosis, spondylitis, spondylolisthesis, osteoporosis, without incurring further hospital-based delays to achieve x-rays on the day of outpatient consultation.

- Basic blood tests prior to referral are also very helpful in saving hospital outpatient time.

BACK PAIN – GENERAL

Introduction

- There is no entirely satisfactory definition of pain. One wise definition describes pain as: "... an unpleasant sensory and emotional experience associated with actual or potential tissue damage ***or described in terms of such damage***" (International Association for the Study of Pain, 1979).
- This definition highlights the fact that pain is very much a problem of individual perception but also avoids describing the frustrating inability of the sufferer to convey to others the ego-destructive unpleasantness of the experience.
- If pain is a problem of perception, each patient's experience of pain constitutes their reality: we cannot deny someone else's pain, as sceptical as we may feel on occasion, and it serves nothing to express such a denial.
- Pain cannot be measured directly; only indirectly by reference to its effect on daily life and the patient's subjective description (see OSWESTRY DISABILITY INDEX).
- Most of us assume that pain is the result of a stimulus to our tissues and the stimulus is causing us damage. "Pain is there for a purpose". This is the Cartesian model of pain (Rene Descartes 1596-1650, French philosopher, mathematician, physiologist). The apparent logic of this model is false when it comes to back pain: any damage beyond mere ageing is rare.
- The same applies to chronic pain, where the original stimulus (back strain injury?) is no longer relevant.
- In any event, back strain injuries can seldom be demonstrated by any test or investigation of any kind.
- There is no single "pain centre" in the brain, but a vast mesh of interconnected areas known as the pain matrix, beautifully demonstrated by PET scanning. *Jones AKP et al. Proc Roy Soc B 1991, 244:39-44.*

Most of the points which follow are repeated under BACK PAIN – LOW because it is considered important there, for those who may avoid them here.

Back Pain – General

1. Back pain is the most common symptom in all of spinal disorders and also the most distressing and frustrating, for patients <u>and</u> doctors. Back pain is a symptom and not a disease although it may present as a symptom of a spinal disease. As it happens, back pain is commonly present *without* any sign of disease, clinically or radiologically. Certainly, it is frequently found together with lumbar **spondylosis** but spondylosis is nothing more than radiological evidence of ageing. It is a philosophical point as to whether ageing is a natural and inevitable process or a disease. The conundrum is further complicated by the fact that spondylosis is a frequent incidental finding in patients who have no back pain.

2. It is also the case that both patients and doctors forget that a great mass of soft tissue (ligaments, intervertebral discs, and muscles) supports the spine, especially at that focus of high physical stress, the lumbosacral junction. Strain injury of these soft tissues occurs frequently as part of daily life. The pain can be as refractory as that for "tennis elbow" (which is presumed also to result from a ligament strain), and neither condition can be visualised by any known method of imaging. While there is full acceptance of the existence of tennis elbow, there is inadequate recognition of the possibility of an equivalent in the spine.

3. All tissues in and around the spine, including the blood vessels in bone, have nerves and nerve endings which can transmit the sensation of pain. The only tissues exempt are the articular cartilage of facet joints and the nucleus plus some inner anular layers of the normal intervertebral disc. In the aged and degenerate disc, even this inner sanctum will be invaded by blood vessels and accompanying nerves.

4. Back pain is a problem as much because of cultural attitudes and mythology, as because of the unpleasantness of the pain itself. It is part of western culture that "pain is there for a purpose: to warn us of damage being done" and "listen to your body: it will tell you what you can do safely". Health professionals frequently reinforce these aphorisms inappropriately, adding to patients' worst fears when there is little to fear other than the pain itself. Then there is the mythology of the wheelchair and the implication of paralysis, as powerful as ever and also perpetuated by well-meaning professionals every day, in the absence of any evidence of serious pathology: "… if you carry on like this you will end up in a wheelchair!".

In the vast majority of patients the ongoing pain is not a sign of progressive damage: the pain serves no purpose except to damage quality of life.

5. The back pain problem is further bedevilled by semantics. Many patients have such intense back pain that some pain is felt in a lower limb ("referred" or "overflow" pain). In the practise of some doctors, any lower limb pain is automatically labelled as "**sciatica**" as a matter of course and thought to show advanced learning. Even the back pain may be labelled "sciatica", erroneously. By old custom, "sciatica" implies nerve root compression and the evidence could be found quite easily on clinical examination, to be confirmed later by MRI. **Back pain alone is almost never caused by neural compression. The matter is important because the beginning of success in diagnosis lies in separating primary back pain from primary lower limb pain, based on where the pain is most severe.** (See Back Pain Algorithm p. 23).

Intense neck pain can be referred in like manner to one or both upper limbs without any cervical nerve root compression to be found in the cervical spine.

6. Most low back pain patients will give one of two contrasting stories about the nature of their pain. The majority will present with the expected story of pain aggravated by physical activity and relieved by rest ("back strain"). A large minority will describe pain unexpectedly aggravated by rest and relieved by gentle movement ("facet arthrosis"). The latter syndrome is so called because it is very like that of patients suffering arthrosis of synovial joints elsewhere: the facet joints are the synovial joints of the spine. The importance of this distinction is the need to recognise that these patients who suffer more pain at rest are not malingerers: not every pain in human experience is necessarily relieved by rest.

7. Chronic pain is the greatest mystery and challenge in all of back pain. There is no easy definition, but all agree that duration of suffering comes into a definition somewhere. Whether this duration should be 3 months or 6 months or 12 months is somewhat beside the point. The unfortunate common experience is that there is no cure for chronic pain, in the absence of clearly treatable underlying pathology.

Back Pain – General

On the other hand, capability in daily life can be restored by engagement in a programme which combines physical training with cognitive behavioural therapy (see FUNCTIONAL RESTORATION).

"I have always been puzzled by the meaning of this phrase (chronic pain) **as distinct from intractable pain. Does it mean that there is a group of patients with tractable pains who never had access to a competent doctor? Does it mean that some patients progress through a treatable stage which is neglected and then later evolve into a perpetual intractable state? Or does it mean that the prolonged experience of pain can itself induce a separate and independent irreversible psychopathological state?** Patrick Wall in Textbook of Pain, 3rd Edition 1994, eds Patrick D Wall, Ronald Melzack. Churchill Livingstone, Edinburgh.

Experimental work has shown that nerve fibres mediating pain sensation can form circular circuits, suggesting a possible mechanism for perpetual pain experience without further external stimulation.
Woolf CJ, Doubell TP. Curr Opin Neurobiol 1994, 4:525-34.

Medications and machines may offer some ease for a time, beyond which the machines fail and the medications produce serious side effects. The best hope for a patient with chronic and disabling low back pain without significant pathology, is a form of cognitive behavioural therapy: FUNCTIONAL RESTORATION. This therapy offers the chance of useful coping rather than cure.

8. Grading pain according to its response to standard analgesics is a recordable measure of perceived severity for that patient at that moment. The OSWESTRY DISABILITY INDEX has 6 grades, serving its own particular purpose. A widely accepted simpler scheme has 4 grades for common clerking purposes:-
    1. No analgesics required. Mild to moderate pain:
    2. Analgesics required: pain abolished, for a time at least.
    3. Analgesics required: pain reduced but still present.
    4. Analgesics used but no improvement in pain.

BACK PAIN – HIGH

1. Implies pain in thoracic spine area identified as "interscapular": between the shoulder blades.
2. Frequent complaint in middle-aged women: gender preference unexplained.
3. Archaic term = "fibrositis": apt because non-threatening.
4. Frequently associated with nodules of muscle in spasm and which can be massaged away.
5. Threatening pathology (cancer, infection, osteoporosis, inflammatory disease) = rare.

Anatomy
- Common sources of pain are presumed to lie in the vast soft tissue anatomy of the dorsal thoracic area, as for lumbar spine and low back pain.
- Mainly muscle and ligament trigger points of uncertain origin: "bad luck" rather than bad injury. **A trigger point is a markedly tender soft tissue focus of consistent location during examination, presumed to lie somewhere in muscle and/or ligament, and which represents nuisance rather than disease.**
- Upper thoracic muscle trigger points = trapezius and rhomboids; mid- and lower thoracic = trapezius, latissimus dorsi, serratus.
- Trigger points in thoracic midline and medial edge of scapula = ligamentous.
- Rare sources of pain: - scapulo-thoracic articulation especially over rib hump of scoliosis;
  - girdle pain of herpes ZOSTER, and intercostal nerve compression in osteoporotic vertebral crush;
  - vertebrae in metastatic disease, infection, ankylosing spondylitis, rheumatoid arthritis, osteoporotic vertebral compression fracture; lung and pleural cancer or infection;
  - neuralgic amytrophy: sudden onset severe muscle pain and atrophy, cause unknown.

Management
- Question for red flags of serious disease: weight loss, loss of appetite, night pain, recent kyphosis deformity, rigors, fever, intractable cough, girdle pain, altered gait, incontinence, perineal numbness.

Back Pain – High

If no red flags:-
- 3 - 6 weeks: expectant observation; standard analgesics if necessary.
- 6 -12 weeks: plain x-ray thoracic spine and chest : routine bloods including full blood count, ESR, uric acid, protein electrophoresis, RA.
- If no abnormality, give standard analgesics and physiotherapy especially deep massage.
- 12 weeks plus: if no adequate response, offer local infiltration of trigger points with mix of triamcinolone 40mg/ml (1 ml) plus Marcaine 0.5% and lignocaine 1%.
- 12 weeks plus: further investigations via MRI and radio-isotope bone scan. Consider referral to specialist.

If all investigations negative:-
- Patient to accept chronicity but with assurances that there is no spinal disease.

If positive or suspect findings:-
- Pursue investigations through to diagnosis, if necessary via biopsy, and treatment of specific disease.

BACK PAIN - LOW

Introduction
Because of our seriously incomplete understanding of this pervasive symptom, it is necessary to make some preliminary statements. Patience in examining these statements will bring its own reward.

1. Low back pain is the most common symptom in all of spinal disorders and also the most distressing, frustrating (for patients <u>and</u> doctors); and the most disabling. Back pain is a symptom and not a disease although it may present as a symptom of a spinal disease. As it happens, back pain is commonly present *without* any sign of disease, clinically or radiologically. Certainly, it is frequently found together with lumbar **spondylosis** but spondylosis is nothing more than radiological evidence of ageing. It is a philosophical point as to whether ageing is a natural and inevitable process or a disease.

2. It is also the case that both patients and doctors forget that a great mass of soft tissue (ligaments, intervertebral discs, and muscles) supports the lumbar spine, especially at that focus of high physical stress, the lumbosacral junction. Strain injury of these soft tissues occurs frequently as part of daily life. The pain can be as refractory as that for "tennis elbow" (which is presumed also to result from a ligament strain), and neither condition can be visualised by any known method of imaging. *While there is full acceptance of the existence of tennis elbow, there is inadequate recognition of the possibility of an equivalent in the spine.*

3. All tissues in and around the spine, including the blood vessels in bone, have nerves and nerve endings which can transmit the sensation of pain. The only tissues exempt are the articular cartilage of facet joints and the nucleus of the normal intervertebral disc. In the aged and degenerate disc, even this inner sanctum will be invaded by blood vessels and accompanying nerves.

4. Back pain is a problem as much because of cultural attitudes and mythology, as because of the unpleasantness of the pain itself. It is part of western culture that "pain is there for a purpose: to warn us of damage being done" and "listen to your body: it will tell you what you can do safely".

Health professionals frequently reinforce these aphorisms inappropriately, adding to patients' worst fears when there is little to fear other than the pain itself. Then there is the mythology of the wheelchair and the implication of paralysis, as powerful as ever and also perpetuated by well-meaning professionals every day, in the absence of any evidence of serious pathology: "... if you carry on like this you will end up in a wheelchair!". **In the vast majority of patients the ongoing pain is not a sign of progressive damage: the pain serves no purpose except to damage quality of life.**

5. The back pain problem is further bedevilled by semantics. Many patients have such intense back pain that some pain is felt in a lower limb ("referred" or "overflow" pain). In the practise of some doctors, any lower limb pain is automatically labelled as "**sciatica**" as a matter of course and thought to show advanced learning. By old custom, "sciatica" implies nerve root compression and the evidence could be found quite easily on clinical examination, to be confirmed later by MRI. Even the back pain may be labelled "sciatica".
Back pain alone is almost never caused by nerve root compression.
The matter is important because the beginning of success in diagnosis lies in separating primary back pain from primary lower limb pain, based on where the pain is most severe.
Another common low back pain referral pattern which can confuse, is pain spreading into the groin and anterior thigh (and testicles in men; labia in women) causing severe distress and embarrassment. This pattern has nothing to do with dermatomes, but it will raise the need to exclude other causes of groin and anterior thigh pain: hip arthritis; femoral hernia; lymphadenopathy; **meralgia paraesthetica**; midlumbar disc prolapse with nerve root compression.

6. Most low back pain patients will give one of two contrasting stories about the nature of their pain. The majority will present with the expected story of pain aggravated by physical activity and relieved by rest ("back strain"). A large minority will describe pain unexpectedly aggravated by rest and relieved by gentle movement ("facet arthrosis"). The latter syndrome is so called because it is very like that of patients suffering arthrosis of synovial joints elsewhere: the facet joints are the synovial joints of the spine. The importance of this distinction is the need to recognise that these patients who suffer more pain at rest are not malingerers: not every pain in human experience is necessarily relieved by rest.

7. Listen out for the "locked back" attack: sudden and crippling back pain with intense immobilising muscle spasm following perfectly innocent postures or movements, requiring days or weeks of unavoidable confinement in bed. Usually superimposed on a long history of chronic back pain of "strain" type (see 6, above). Description is consistent from patient to patient and perfectly genuine. Mechanism not known.

Diagnosis (see BACK PAIN - ALGORITHM).
- **The vast majority of back pain is of nuisance value only, even if the nuisance is considerable.**
- Diagnostic methods are increased in stages, depending on the duration and severity of the symptoms, and always with the "red flag" symptoms and signs in mind, where their presence may indicate a serious underlying disease after all.
- The **first step** is to seek clarity from the patient, through careful questioning, as to whether the symptoms are maximal in the **low back** area or in the **lower limb**. If the latter, we may be dealing with a nerve root compression which will need a diagnostic and therapeutic approach rather different from that which would apply to common low back pain.
- The **second step** requires us to deal with **"red flags"** ie those symptoms and signs which suggest some uncommon but far more serious disease eg cancer, infection, lower limb weakness and perineal sphincter paralysis, and arterial obstructive disease.
- Ask about weight loss, loss of appetite, night pain, rigors, sweats, perineal and peri-anal sensation, bladder and bowel control.
- Assess peripheral lower limb pulses in every patient, as a matter of habit.

Management
- The algorithm (p.23) is self-explanatory. In the absence of "red flags" the first requirement is reassurance for the great majority of patients.
- Prescribe a combination of standard analgesics and/or anti-inflammatories plus any favoured set of gentle exercises. Bed rest only for short periods of intractable pain. Local infiltration for focal trigger points (see "Treatment" below).

Back Pain – Low

- For "locked back": home visits for once daily intramuscular pethidine and anti-inflammatory eg Mobiflex 20 mg, for 2 – 3 days.
- Refer to specialist when primary treatments finally fail and symptoms produce disability for the activities of daily living.
- Referral to spine surgeon should be more urgent for "red flags", and also in suspected nerve root compression for the simple reason that the pain of nerve root compression is frequently unendurable.
- Referral should include a basic set of plain x-rays of lumbar spine and pelvis, to enable the surgeon to exclude some obvious explanatory pathology eg infiltrative disease, spondylosis, spondylitis, spondylolisthesis, osteoporosis, without incurring further hospital-based delays to achieve x-rays on the day of outpatient consultation.
- Basic blood tests prior to referral are also very helpful.

Treatment
- as described here is for the pain and not any serious underlying condition.
- is applied in graduated stages of invasiveness, beginning with strenuous reassurance, standard analgesics and anti-inflammatory medications, even in combination. Narcotic medications in any form are intended only for short term crises of pain.
- Physiotherapy, osteopathy, and chiropractic gentle manipulation techniques are most likely to succeed in patients with "facet arthrosis" pain.
- Soft tissue "trigger points" lend themselves to temporary relief for up to 3 months, by local infiltration with large volume local anaesthetic and small volume steroid in combination.
- Local infiltration is a largely lost skill in primary care. The vast majority of trigger points are found on the iliac crests or over the lumbosacral facet joints. ***Injection into the most tender focus by fine needle up to 3 cms depth is quite safe in an adult. The infiltrate is a combination of: 10 ml Marcaine 0.5%, 5 ml Lignocaine 1%, and Triamcinolone 40mg in 1ml.***

- Surgery in the form of spinal fusion (arthrodesis) is a final therapy of desperation, but remains the most successful treatment for refractory and intractable back pain.
- "Instability" **IS NOT AN INDICATION FOR FUSION SURGERY** except possibly after major spinal injury: the concept is hopelessly confused, and does not necessarily have any relationship to the acceptable indication, namely, intractable and disabling low back pain with demonstrable abnormalities in only one or two adjacent segments.
- Segmental levels to be grafted are determined by MRI. Spinal fusion of more than two adjacent segmental levels carries a high failure rate through pseudarthrosis.
- Post-operative rehabilitation is a slow progression of physical capability but excludes all heavy lifting and strenuous physical stress for at least 12 months. Walking is beneficial from start: excellent and underrated. No driving for first two months. Spinal brace/corset for heavy or hyperactive patients, for 3-4 months.
- Surgical success judged no sooner than 12–18 months post-operatively: major gratifying reduction in pain and plain x-rays suggesting bone graft consolidation.
- Newer procedures avoiding need for bone grafting are intended to allow residual segmental motion. They depend on long lasting integrity of implants without fusion, (unlikely) eg pedicle screws attached to cables; various metal and high density polyethylene disc replacements.
- On recovery from a severe attack of back pain, common sense would dictate against a return to physically strenuous occupations and hobbies for those whose pain was aggravated by physical effort initially. The same advice applies to all those recovering from spinal fusion surgery, for at least 12 months.

CANCER
[See Tumour p.181]

CAUDA EQUINA SYNDROME

- One of only two surgical emergencies in spinal disorders. (The other is EPIDURAL ABSCESS; spinal injury requires urgent treatment but is not a surgical emergency).
- Is a spectrum of symptoms and signs (rather than a single clear entity) of impending or developed lower motor neuron deficit involving both lower limbs and perineum.
- **Cause** = almost always a large lumbar central disc prolapse.

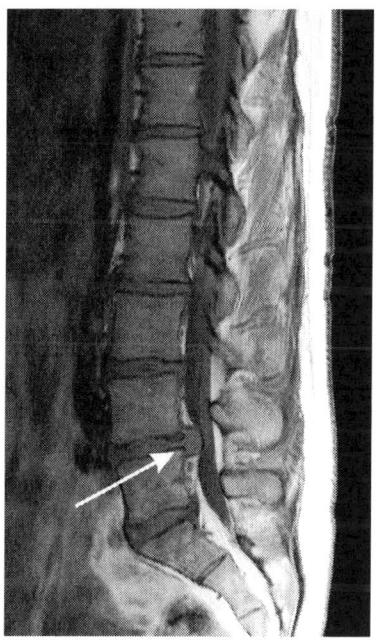

Large central disc prolapse, L4-5 (arrowed) producing cauda equina compression.

Cauda Equina Syndrome

- **Presentation** = History of some or all of: **RED FLAGS:** bilateral sciatica, lower limb weakness and numbness, perineal numbness and varying degrees of urinary/faecal incontinence.
- **Examination:** some or all of: **RED FLAGS:** reduced perineal sensation, diminished knee/ankle tendon reflexes and demonstrable lower limb power loss, patulous anus, overflow urinary incontinence.
- **Diagnosis** = **HIGH INDEX OF SUSPICION** followed by emergency MRI.
- **Treatment** = urinary catheter; pain control; emergency decompression via laminotomy, bilateral if necessary.
- **Prognosis** = poor for sphincter recovery.
- **Controversy** = whether there is a saving of neurological deficit if decompression performed within hours of diagnosis, even in early hours of morning, as against elective "next day" surgery.
- Expensive medico-legal cases continue to feature a serious lack of suspicion coupled with a total absence of clinical examination.
- If investigations (MRI/myelography) fail to reveal any significant neural compression, consider rare medical conditions which can mimic a cauda equina syndrome: myasthenia gravis; mulitple sclerosis.

COCCYX and COCCYDYNIA

Neglected distal termination of spine, usually 4 vestigial vertebral body segments variously segmented or not at all segmented. Overall shape is that of a bony V without any neural canal, articulating with distal end of the sacrum by a combination of small synovial joints and a vestigial intervertebral disc.
Too frequently dismissed source of disabling pain (coccydynia) in some patients. Usually spontaneous onset. Occasional history of direct trauma as in hard fall onto buttocks on ice or down stairs; or indirect trauma of childbirth. Females are usual sufferers. Source of pain still not known but may be multiple: sacrococcygeal joint/disc strain and/or ligamentous strain at insertion of pelvic floor ("tennis elbow" of the coccyx?). (See also p.16).

History reveals patients who prefer to stand; cannot drive long distance; change sitting position frequently, from one buttock to other; little relief from analgesics; affects every aspect of daily living. Pain aggravated by passage of constipated stool.

Examination reveals marked tenderness in region of sacrococcygeal joint, aggravated by pressure on distal coccyx. Bimanual palpation seldom necessary to elicit typical pain but worthwhile to exclude rectal mass.

Investigations of little use. Plain x ray confirms only what we know from pelvic imaging in those who have no coccydynia: that the coccyx can take up a variety of positions as normal, without revealing pathology. <u>MRI is essential to exclude intra-pelvic pathology.</u> Histology of excised sacrococcygeal joints revealed variable moderate degeneration of articular cartilage or disc.

Treatment beyond mere reassurance and analgesia implies surgical excision (coccygectomy). Local infiltration with steroid and local anaesthetic alongside coccyx margins is seldom successful for more than days or weeks. Coccygectomy will provide gratifying long term relief in 70% of patients. Risks are rectal perforation during surgery (extremely rare) and wound infection (surprisingly rare). Surgical technique requires careful subperiosteal excision and little more.

Coccygectomy for coccydynia: case series and review of literature. Balain B, Eisenstein S et al. Spine 31:E414-20, 2006.
Coccydynia. Review article. Nathan ST et al. J Bone Joint Surg (B) 92-B:1622-7, 2010.

COMPLEMENTARY THERAPIES

    Acupuncture   Meditation
    Aromatherapy   Osteopathy
    Chiropractic   Reflexology
    Chondroitin sulphate   Reiki
    Herbal remedies   Yoga
    Homeopathy

Syn: Alternative (less kind); Unorthodox (unkind); Non-orthodox (still unkind).

Are therapeutic methods, techniques, medications, and philosophies generally considered not mainstream therapies supposedly on the basis that there is insufficient foundation in science to justify these therapies.

Historically there was serious antipathy against such therapies on the part of the "orthodox" profession because of an expectation that life threatening or limb threatening diseases could not be treated, and persistence with the unorthodox would hasten death or destruction. This prejudice was inevitably combined with some professional jealousy and the conviction that complementary therapists were not subject to training and examination of equal rigour to the orthodox, nor equally monitored in practise. Not only was there some hypocrisy in this (most modern medications began as herbal remedies without any understanding of the chemistry of the active ingredient), but there was a general disregard of the fact that these therapies were frequently successful in treating painful musculoskeletal conditions.

Much has changed the climate of mutual antagonism: some complementary therapies have been tested in large "orthodox" trials and found to be successful ("whatever works for the patient, works"); there is far less fear of professional competition; and complementary therapies have been supported by members of the royal family. Many doctors trained in orthodox schools offer complementary therapies after appropriate training. Complementary therapists now have a highly developed sense of when to recommend specialist opinion.

Chiropractic, osteopathy, and acupuncture have become part of mainstream musculoskeletal medical practice.

COMPLICATIONS

1. Death
2. Paralysis
3. CSF leak
4. Infection
5. Thrombosis
6. Pseudarthrosis
7. Donor site problems
8. Recurrent disc prolapse
9. Wound problems
10. Implant problems
11. Expectations dashed

A surgical complication is an adverse unintended physical or perceived harm occurring in the peri-operative period, whether the result of a surgical error or of sheer misfortune.

No surgery is without complications at one time or another. Doctors do not need to be told that, but patients do. Patients being offered surgery are frequently visibly surprised to receive this information. Doctors continue to wonder at such naivety. We must remember that the experience of surgery for most patients is appendicectomy or tonsillectomy in childhood. These operations are very nearly 100% successful; no residual pain, paralysis, or deformity. **Most of the complications of spinal surgery are potentially extremely serious but also very rare.** Listing these complications for the patient facing surgery is a requirement of the modern consenting process. (See also CONSENT). Rarity of the more serious complications should be emphasised, but patients need to be made aware nevertheless, in order to be able to take some responsibility for the surgical treatment plan.

Patients need to be reminded strenuously and repeatedly of the "Three Laws of Eisenstein" in respect of surgery for spinal disorders:-
1. There is **no cure** (of all pain, comparable to surgery for appendicitis, for instance).
2. There is **no guarantee** (of "success").
3. And **no patient has to have an operation**.

Complications

General:

VARIOUS DECOMPRESSION PROCEDURES *Risk of at least one major complication is **1.6%**.*
    Ramirez LF, Thisted R. Neurosurgery 1989, 25:226-30.

LUMBAR DISCECTOMY *Risk of all complications is **8.7% (first surgery)**: dural perforation, neural damage, deep vein thrombosis, pulmonary embolus, discitis, urinary tract infection (no death). Risk of all complications is **19.1% (revision surgery)**: ditto*
    Morgan-Hough CV, Jones PW, Eisenstein SM. J Bone Joint Surg Br 2003, 85:871-4.

Specific:

1. **Death** Extremely rare. Intra-operative = anaesthetic related or uncontrollable haemorrhage from a major vessel during anterior procedures. Post-operative = pulmonary embolus = more common than vascular injury but still highly unusual thanks to routine prophylaxis for deep vein thrombosis. Also septicaemia and myocardial infarction.
Risk within first 30 days (for various lumbar decompression procedures) is 1/2000 operations (0.05%).
    Jansson KA et al. J Bone Joint Surg Br 2004, 86:841-7.
    Ramirez LF, Thisted R. Neurosurgery 1989, 25:226-30.

2. **Paralysis** Extremely rare, despite frequency of surgery right down to dura of spinal cord or cauda equina. Most likely to consist of weakness of action at the ankle joint following decompression surgery for lumbar disc prolapse, during which some inadvertent nerve damage took place. Less frequent but more devastating is paraplegia associated with scoliosis correction. Spinal cord monitoring of electrical function of the cord is routine during scoliosis surgery and gives early warning of spinal cord distress. Even less frequent, thankfully, is quadriplegia associated with cervical cord damage during neck surgery.

Recurrent laryngeal nerve palsy with hoarse soft voice, after anterior cervical surgery, qualifies as "paralysis". Vast majority are temporary.

Complications

ANTERIOR CERVICAL FUSION Risk of permanent recurrent laryngeal nerve palsy is **0.3%**.
 Risk of temporary recurrent laryngeal nerve palsy, provided ET cuff pressure eased during tracheal retraction in anterior cervical fusion is **1.7%**.
 Apfelbaum RI et al. Spine 2000, 25:2906-12.

ANTERIOR THORACIC AND LUMBAR SPINE FUSIONS AS FOR SCOLIOSIS Risk of cord or cauda equina paralysis is **0.2%** (2/1000).
 Faciszewski T et al. Spine 1995, 20:1592-9.

SCOLIOSIS SURGERY Risk of cord or cauda equina paralysis is **0.55%** (5.5/1000).
 Delank KS et al. Arch Orthop Trauma Surg 2005, 125: 33-41.

ADULT SPINAL DEFORMITY CORRECTION AND FUSION
 Risk of lumbar nerve root palsy is **1.4% (first surgery)**.
 Risk of lumbar nerve root palsy is **3.8% (revision surgery)**. Pateder DB, Kostuik JP Spine 2005, 30:1632-6.

LUMBAR DISCECTOMY
 Risk of nerve root injury is **0.4%**.
 Morgan-Hough CV, Jones PW, Eisenstein SM. J Bone Joint Surg Br 2003, 85:871-4.

3. **Cerebrospinal Fluid (CSF) leak** Probably the most common complication of decompression operations, resulting from a defect in the meningeal (dural) covering of the nerve roots, created inadvertently despite the greatest care. Usually without damage to the nerve. Rarely produces a troublesome swelling under the skin which may require separate surgical repair. Beware of any surgeon who claims never to have created a CSF leak.

LUMBAR DISCECTOMY
 Risk of dural perforation is **5.5%**.
 Morgan-Hough CV, Jones PW, Eisenstein SM. J Bone Joint Surg Br 2003, 85:871-4.

Complications

4 . **Infection**   Most likely originating elsewhere within the patient from some cryptic asymptomatic source (ear? tooth?) or contamination from ward or theatre environment. Organism most likely = Staphylococcus aureus, especially methicillin resistant variety (MRSA). Less common but potentially lethal is Clostridium Difficile ("C diff"). Infection more common in general hospitals than in elective specialty hospitals. Protracted periods of tissue retraction during spinal surgery may predispose to postoperative wound infection. Diabetes constitutes highest independent risk *(Olsen MA, Nepple JJ, Riew KD et al. J Bone Joint Surg Am 2008, 90:62-9).* Prophylaxis in practice consists of laminar flow ventilation in theatre; pre-operative broad spectrum antibiotics; antibiotic wound washout at frequent intervals. Effectiveness of these measures probably not quantified.

SURGICAL SITE OVERALL   Risk is **2.0%**
Olsen MA, Nepple JJ, Riew KD et al. J Bone Joint Surg Am 2008, 90:62-9.

ANTERIOR SPINAL FUSION   Risk of deep wound infection is **0.6%**

Faciszewski T et al. Spine 1995, 20:1592-9.

LUMBAR DISCECTOMY   Risk of disc space infection is **0.2%.**
Risk of urinary tract infection is **0.9%.**
Morgan-Hough CV, Jones PW, Eisenstein SM. J Bone Joint Surg Br 2003, 85:871-4.

5. **Thrombosis**   Blood clotting in the deep veins of calf, thigh, and/or pelvis probably occurs more frequently than we know through symptoms. Painful swollen lower limbs discovered in the days following surgery, should trigger investigations by venography or Doppler scanning to exclude or confirm thrombosis. Treatment is necessary for its own sake, but especially to prevent clot travelling to lung and causing a potentially fatal pulmonary embolus.

POSTERIOR LUMBAR DECOMPRESSIONS OR FUSIONS   Risk of DVT is **2%** *(all in elastic stockings:* **0% with pneumatic compression**).
Ferree BA, Wright AM. Spine 1993, 18:1079-82.

LUMBAR DISCECTOMY   Risk of DVT is **0.4%.**
Risk of pulmonary embolus is **0.4%.**
Morgan-Hough CV, Jones PW, Eisenstein SM. J Bone Joint Surg Br 2003, 85:871-4.

Complications

6. **Pseudarthrosis** Persistent back pain after spinal fusion surgery can have several origins but the most likely is failure of the bone transplant (graft) to consolidate across all relevant intervertebral segments. By universal convention, a lumbar fusion should be given 12 to 18 months to prove itself, and a cervical fusion 2 to 3 months, irrespective of technique. (See also p.124)
*Risk is close to **100%** if using cadaver bone.*
   Herron LD, Newman MH. Spine 1989, 16:496-500.

*Risk is **6%** using autogenous fibular dowel grafts in dysplastic spondylolisthesis.*
   Hanson DS et al. Spine 2002, 15:1982-8.

Apart from these two specialised situations, the general risk of pseudarthrosis is not known because the available non-invasive imaging techniques are inadequate for discovering the absolute incidence of graft failure. A fair estimate would place the risk of symptomatic pseudarthrosis at **5%-10%,** for lumbar fusions of all kinds. Risk is far less for thoracic and cervical fusions.

7. **Donor site** Pain; scar. At this time (2012) there is not yet a bone graft substitute to match the qualities of autogenous bone, harvested usually from one or both iliac blades. Bone graft is necessary for spinal arthrodesis ("fusion") surgery. The harvest (donor) site can be the source of chronic pain after surgery, and of such severity as to ruin the possibly good result of pain relief in the spine itself. The cause of this donor site pain is uncertain, but very likely related to a combination of: extent of dissection; periosteal stripping; injury to cluneal nerves and others running just below the iliac crest; untrimmed sharp corners left after graft removal.
*Risk of chronic donor site pain is **25%**.*
   Summers BN, Eisenstein SM. J Bone Joint Surg (Br) 71-B: 677-80, 1989.

8. **Recurrent disc prolapse** On average, one in ten post-discectomy patients will return with some degree of recurrence of sciatica within the first five to ten years, and the cause will be found to be a recurrent disc prolapse. Probably amenable to repeat surgery, but with an increase in all the complications implicit in repeat surgery: dural tear; nerve injury; persistent sciatica; post-discectomy back pain. The cause of recurrence is bad luck rather than bad surgery: some disc fragment previously well anchored, has come adrift and found its way into the spinal canal.

Complications

*Risk of recurrence in two recent studies is **8%**.*
> Cinotti G et al. J Bone Joint Surg [Br] 1998, 80-B:825-32.
> Morgan-Hough CVJ et al. J Bone Joint Surg [Br] 2003, 85-B: 871-4.

*Risk of recurrence within one year is **1%**.*
> Wera GD et al. J Bone Joint Surg [Am] 2008, 90:10-5.

Mean interval between primary surgery and symptomatic recurrence is 7 years.

9. **Wound** Pain, cosmesis, incisional hernia, incisional haematoma, cerebrospinal fluid leak.
*Risk of incisional haematoma (variety of lumbar decompressions) = **8-9/10,000** operations.*
> Ramirez LF Thisted R. Neurosurgery 1989, 25:226-30.

10. **Implant** loosening, breakage, misplacement, displacement, infection, neural injury. Applies mainly to stabilisation operations, seldom performed now without some kind of supportive or replacement implant. Not always symptomatic. Literature is vast for each type of implant. Complications with increasing difficulty of insertion: pedicle screws, cages, disc replacements. Late pain in solid fusion may be caused by metal implants for reasons not understood.
*Risks with PLIF threaded cage: dural laceration = **15%**; persistent back pain = **15%**; pseudarthrosis = **15%**; migration = **3%**.*
> Elias WJ et al. J Neurosurg 2000, 93:45-52.

*Risks with pedicle screws: overall = **54%**; deep infection = **5%**; misplacement = **6.5%**; breakage = **12%**.*
> Jutte PC, Castelein RM. Eur Spine J 2002, 11:594-8.

11. **Expectations dashed** Much spinal surgery is intended to mitigate pain. Expectations are always likely to be somewhat unrealistic in this age of medical miracles. Despite repeated warnings to patients in preparation for surgery, unmet expectations probably constitute the single largest category of failure.
Level of risk probably not capable of calculation.

CONSENT

The ancient Hippocratic tradition implied a contract established between patient and doctor by the mere act of the patient arriving at the doctor's premises seeking help. The contract was unwritten: the doctor would do his utmost for the patient and the patient would trust the doctor's expertise and best intentions without demur. The doctor would be rewarded by the patient, within the patient's capacity, or go unrewarded if necessary.

This picture of a doctor/patient relationship is so far from current experience as to beggar belief that it ever existed except in the minds of nostalgic dreamers. It is with difficulty that we have to be reminded that it existed pretty well intact until mid-20th century. A massive culture shift throughout the western world, with state provision of health care out of taxation, resulted in a mutual loss of trust between patient and doctor. A hopelessly unrealistic expectation on the part of the public, of perfection in all things, has seen the emergence of pervasive personal injury litigation for outcomes short of the expected perfection.

Doctors, especially surgeons, and the hospitals in which they work have had to counter the frequent charge in court that the patient/claimant had not been adequately informed of the potential complications of the surgery performed (see COMPLICATIONS). The claim would be that adequate information would have resulted in the patient's refusal to undergo the surgery on offer. "Adequately informed" is now the requirement before surgery, better known as "informed consent". The process requires detailed information on possible complications, as well as details of the operation intended. Documentation of the consenting procedure is necessary if the consent achieved is to be useful in fending off litigation. The process is understandably tedious and time consuming for surgeons, and the task cannot be delegated. The information is frequently beyond the understanding of the patient; beyond the capacity of many patients to retain in memory; and sometimes sufficiently frightening as to result in a refusal by the patient to proceed.

There is some good to be found in this loss of innocence and trust in modern surgical life. Surgeons are forced repeatedly to confront their fallibility and the fact that **no one has to have an operation, for anything, ever**. Patients are forced to participate in the decision-making as never before, and it is possible that

Consent

some patients are grateful for this: "Whose body is it, anyway?". For some patients this sharing of responsibility is sharing too much. "You are the doctor, you tell me!!", but the alternative today, too frequently, would be litigation against the surgeon.

Spinal surgery is now considered so dangerous in terms of the likelihood of litigation, that the professional insurance companies have created a special premium category for spinal surgeons alone, higher than "ordinary" orthopaedic and neurosurgeons, but just below that most expensive practise of all, obstetrics.

Consenting for spinal surgery should therefore be robust, conducted preferably by the senior surgeon, preferably in the presence of family witnesses. If patients are scared off by the graphic description of complications possible, then so be it. That is the "patient choice" which modern social and legal cultures have decreed. In the USA, consenting is frequently recorded on video.

The complications of spinal surgery are: death, paralysis (including recurrent laryngeal nerve where relevant), dural tear with CSF leak, infection, thrombosis (leg and lung), implant misplacement and loosening (if relevant), persistence of symptoms, scar pain and cosmesis, pseudarthrosis and donor site pain (in spinal fusions), recurrence of prolapse and spinal stenosis.
The levels of risk are given in COMPLICATIONS.

Where approaches to the spine are to be made through the chest and/or abdomen, the possible (but rare) complications relevant to these approaches should be revealed.

DISABILITY, IMPAIRMENT, INCAPACITY and HANDICAP

Although these words are supposed to represent differing aspects of defective functioning of various organs, the reality is that they are separated by social science definitions only with the greatest difficulty. Their use is well-intentioned: to replace the word "cripple" with all its archaic pejorative overtones. The confusion is not improved when one term is defined in terms of another. The WHO and dictionary definitions illustrate the problem:-

Disability: "Any restriction or lack of ability to perform an activity in a manner ...considered normal for a human being. (It) reflects the consequences of impairment...or defect of one or more organs..." "An impairment or defect of one or more organs or members".

Also the name of a benefit which can be claimed from the DWP in the UK ie Disability Living Allowance (DLA).

Impairment: "Any loss or abnormality of psychologic, physiologic, or anatomic structure or function."

Handicap: "A physical, mental, or emotional condition that interferes with an individual's normal functioning."

Incapacity: (Not listed in Stedman's Medical Dictionary). In the UK, the term is applied to a certain benefit paid out by the DWP to those who qualify on the basis that their defects exclude their ability to enter gainful employment.

These terms are used interchangeably in daily life. There are earnest professionals who seek to impute fine distinctions through narrow definitions. The resulting semantic confusion is unnecessary. "When I use a word it means just what I choose it to mean..." (Humpty Dumpty to Alice: THROUGH THE LOOKING GLASS   Lewis Carroll).

Generally, it may be accepted that an **impairment** (eg lower limb amputation) may produce a **disability** eg slow running with a prosthesis, which may in turn produce a **handicap** depending on specific circumstances e.g. patient was previously an Olympic marathon runner.

Disability, Impairment, Incapacity and Handicap

The subject is important mainly because of common "mechanical" back pain. The indication for surgical fusion should be based primarily on an assessment of disability rather than on some assessment of "disease". Of greater significance is the fact that back pain is the second most expensive condition in the developed world (after the common cold) in terms of days off sick, lost production, and welfare pay-out for long term disability.

DISC

Anatomy [see ANATOMY & PHYSIOLOGY].

Degenerative Disc Disease. Overly dramatic and overused term causing patients unnecessary distress, intended to designate variable disc <u>dehydration</u> and associated osteophytosis (bony overgrowth), otherwise known as "spondylosis" (see SPONDYLOSIS). Usually part of normal ageing process of middle life and beyond, but certainly frequently associated with chronic back pain and neck pain. Sometimes seen well before middle age, representing a possible familial or genetic predisposition as in **Heberden**'s arthropathy, or simply "bad luck". Never "bad disease". Other life-style factors associated with symptomatic spondylosis (and disc prolapse – see below) are heavy physical work, lifting, truck driving, obesity, and smoking.

In terms of numbers of patients, the aged disc is responsible for most of the daily distressing symptoms arising in the lumbar spine: almost universal low back pain; and spinal stenosis with disabling **claudication** in the fit elderly. The ageing disc loses height with loss of water from the nucleus pulposus. The loss of nucleus turgor allows translational movements at disc level between adjacent vertebrae owing to slack ligaments. The loss of nucleus turgor also allows major pressures within the facet joints, with the development of facet joint arthrosis. This can produce the classical synovial joint back pain characterised by pain worse at rest (see BACK PAIN – LOW); and the general osteophytosis can produce classical lumbar stenosis with claudication.

Disc

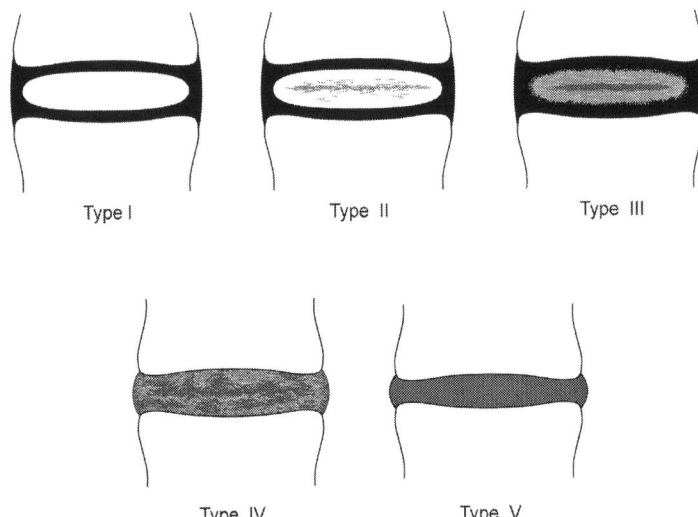

(Magnetic resonance classification of lumbar intervertebral disc degeneration. Pfirrmann CW et al. Spine 26:1873-8, 2001)

Discitis [see DISCITIS]

Disc Prolapse / Herniation /"Slipped disc" Clinical significance is based on the tendency for prolapsed disc material to compress neural tissue ie spinal cord and/ or segmental nerve roots. Vast majority of prolapses are posterolateral, at all levels of the spine, so that the majority of clinical presentations are as unilateral nerve root compression symptoms and signs ("sciatica"). Posterior central prolapses at any level down to the cord termination at L1/L2 may compress spinal cord causing varying degrees of upper motor neurone symptoms and signs (**myelopathy**). Central prolapses further caudal may produce varying degrees of the CAUDA EQUINA syndrome.

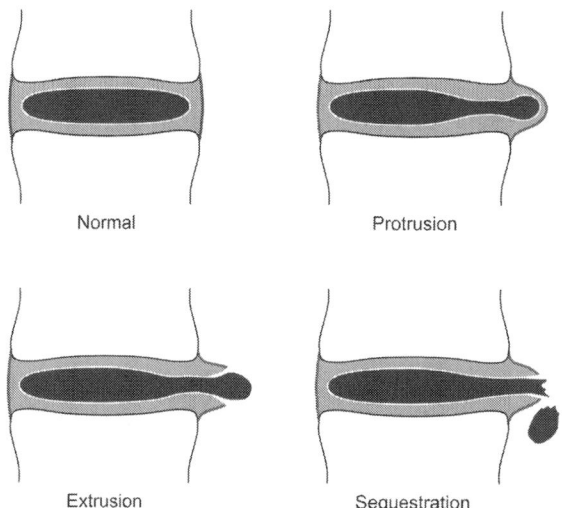

Normal Protrusion Extrusion Sequestration

There are three types of prolapse, identifiable as probable on MRI but requiring confirmation only by direct inspection at surgery :-

Protrusion: the anulus bulges into the spinal canal or root canal, pushed by prolapsing material, but the final layers of anulus remain intact. Implication = unlikely that there will be any free fragments of disc tissue to be found elsewhere in the spinal canal; unlikely that nerve root will be adherent to anulus.

Extrusion: disc material has erupted through a complete defect or tear in the anulus but there are no free fragments of disc to be found elsewhere. Implication = nerve root may be adherent to exposed disc material if inflammatory reaction allowed to mature. Adds to hazards of surgery.

Sequestration: disc material is not only extruded but free fragments have shifted proximally and/or distally to lie behind adjacent vertebral bodies, or deep within the root canal. Implication = there must be a careful search for free fragments during decompression surgery to avoid residual post-operative sciatic symptoms.

Disc

Clinical presentation is that of neural compression, but we know that at any level in the spine, the vastly most common cause of neural compression will be a disc prolapse. The unremitting pain of a particularly severe sciatica is said to be second only to that of an impacted kidney stone.

The most frequent levels for prolapse and consequent nerve root compression will be in the lower **lumbar** spine:

History reveals an episode of back pain, soon replaced by a dramatic and disabling sciatica stretching from buttock to foot, and probably combined with numbness and tingling (paraesthesia) in calf and foot. Pain and paraesthesia along the lateral border of the foot suggest an S1 root compression; on the dorsum of the foot and big toe suggests an L5 root compression.

Examination should reveal a limited straight leg raising on the painful side because this manoeuvre produces an unbearable increase in intensity of sciatic pain. **However, many clinicians allow themselves to be fooled by a straight leg raise limited by back pain only, and only because they forgot to ask the patient which pain is stopping the leg raise.** Plantar flexion weakness with loss of sensation along the lateral border of the foot, and a diminished/absent ankle jerk, suggest an S1 root compression; dorsiflexion weakness ("foot drop") with reduced sensation dorsum of foot, in the presence of normal reflexes, suggest an L5 root compression.

Pain anterior thigh (femoratica) is less common. If combined with reduced sensation anterior thigh, an absent knee jerk, and a positive femoral nerve stretch test, think of mid and upper lumbar nerve root compression.

Disc prolapse in the **thoracic** spine is relatively rare, but far more dangerous for the patient. The first presentation may be that of an upper motor neurone syndrome with advancing spastic paraparesis, possibly combined with segmental nerve symptoms of intercostal neuralgia.

In the **cervical** spine a disc prolapse is most likely to spare the spinal cord but compress a segmental nerve root producing cervical radiculopathy: intractable upper limb pain and paraesthesia in a roughly dermatomal distribution; a positive Spurling test (see EPONYMS); upper limb muscle weakness, and loss of a reflex.

Disc

Investigation is justified if pain and disability remain beyond clinical control after an enthusiastic trial of days of rest and analgesia. It is silly to be dogmatically prescriptive as to how long this trial of conservative treatment should last; each patient must be handled according to their manifest suffering. It must be remembered that other dreadful but rare diseases such as cancer and infection also present with sciatica and there can be no harm in excluding these at an early stage. Advancing neurological deficit will require urgent investigation irrespective of pain.

MRI will reveal all, including the less common "far lateral" disc prolapse which traps a nerve root within or beyond the root canal. Check carefully that the revealed prolapse is found on the same side as the presenting symptoms and signs.

In the *thoracic* spine the MRI is likely to reveal a disc prolapse both central and lateral, with calcified anulus, suggesting a long delay between prolapse and symptoms.

In the *cervical* spine the prolapse is more likely to be seen to compress a cervical nerve root rather than cervical cord, thanks to the large CSF reservoir between disc space and cord.

Plain radiographs of the spine, especially the anteroposterior view, are essential for excluding junctional variation of anatomy (lumbarisation; sacralisation) which in turn may lead the unwary surgeon into operating at the wrong level.

Treatment will always start with analgesia and a period of observation. By the time MRI investigations have been instigated it is likely that a decision will already have been made for surgical nerve root decompression and discectomy (see COMPLICATIONS; CONSENT; SURGERY - DECOMPRESSION).

In the **lumbar** spine the operation is usually performed with the patient prone, knees and hips flexed 90^0, and abdomen free. The level of intended surgery is confirmed by needle marker shown on image intensifier. After a small midline incision of 3 centimetres, the decompression is performed by interlaminar flavectomy, medial facetectomy, laminotomy, careful retraction of the compressed nerve root and finally discectomy itself. The use of an operating microscope is thought helpful by some.

Percutaneous techniques are on the way but are not likely to find wide acceptance until the clarity of visualisation through water/saline can be achieved. Bipolar coagulation of epidural vessels is important prior to closure. Patient is mobilised as soon as possible within the limits of pain.

Disc

In the **thoracic** spine the approach must be anterior: attempting to reach the prolapsed disc posteriorly will probably require a dangerous degree of cord retraction. The anterior approach implies a thoracotomy and careful counting to arrive at the correct segmental level. Careful discectomy, preferably following a vertically extensive dissection involving adjacent parts of vertebral bodies, may yet result in neurological disaster. The pre-operative consent process must include this stark warning. The chest is closed over an intercostal drain and lung inflation checked radiologically. Postoperative recovery after removal of the chest drain is rapid. In the **cervical** spine the approach is usually anterior, again for reasons of access without a need to retract the cord. The patient is supine with cervical spine in some extension. The standard midcervical transverse incision invariably heals very well. Choice of side depends on the preference of the surgeon. Dissection on the right side must be sufficiently careful to avoid damage to the recurrent laryngeal nerve; on the left side the thoracic duct is vulnerable. On both sides the dissection must remain medial to the carotid sheath. The suspected culpable disc is marked by a needle and the level confirmed radiologically in theatre. A careful discectomy is performed with most effort concentrated on the side of neural compression, until it is possible to pass a probe easily into the relevant root canal without hindrance. Opinions differ markedly between surgeons as to the need for use of an operating microscope; the requirement for a fusion of the cleared segment; and, if a fusion is considered necessary, whether the graft material should be autogenous bone or some substitute. Wound closure must always include a wound drain.
Irrespective of differing opinions, patients make a rapid recovery. If a fusion has been performed, a cervical support (collar) is recommended for eight weeks.

DISCITIS

Discitis is a rare cause of spinal pain at any level from neck to low back and of varying intensity depending on underlying pathology. The diagnosis of discitis is made initially on plain x-ray: a characteristic combination of loss of disc height, a very dark bubble of nitrogen gas in the disc space, and irregular "moth-eaten" endplates. The vertebral body cancellous bone adjacent to the endplates may show alternating lysis and sclerosis. Compare with simple dehydration of disc.

Discitis is **infective** or **inflammatory**. Infecting organisms are most likely to be staph aureus or tuberculosis, from infections elsewhere in the patient, and carried in the slow vertebral capillary circulation adjacent to the endplates. A child presenting with a high fever, rigid spine, and severe back pain, almost certainly has pyogenic discitis. Inflammatory discitis may be a component of rheumatoid arthritis or, (ironically) a pseudarthrosis in ankylosing spondylitis.

The plain x-ray appearances are not specific for the different pathologies but early destruction of the disc suggests infections rather than cancer. Additional tests are required: full blood count, ESR, CRP, RA, and needle aspiration of disc if all else fails. Discitis following discography was once thought to be "chemical" but is now known to be infective.

MRI shows high signal on T2 (oedema, inflammation, pus) Radio-isotope bone scan shows a dark black focus which could be metastatic cancer.

Treatment is determined by the causative pathology. Infective discitis is treated by appropriate antibiotics. In tuberculosis, surgery in the form of debridement and fusion would be indicated only if there are complications of an associated vertebral osteomyelitis: intractable pain, advancing neurology, progressive deformity, adjacent soft tissue abscess, antibiotic resistance. Inflammatory discitis will attract medications appropriate to the specific diagnosis. The pseudarthrosis of ankylosing spondylitis may require surgical fusion for intractrable pain.

Discitis

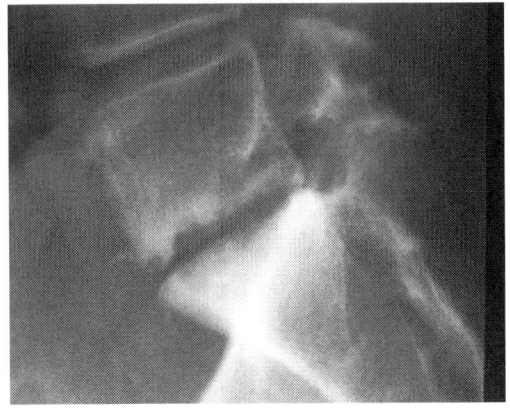

L5-S1 Discitis. Middle aged female. Bacterial infection

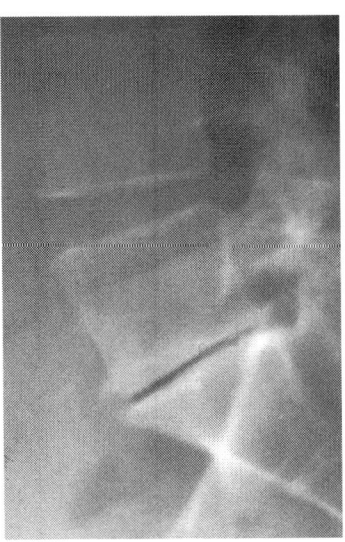

L5-S1 Disc dehydration
in middle-aged female – NOT DISCITIS.

Discitis

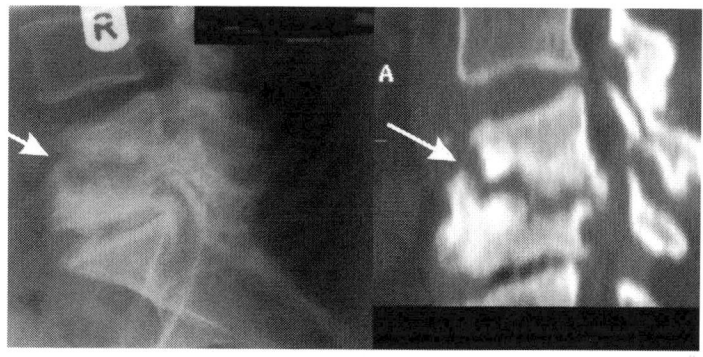

"Bad disc; good news" (rather have infection than cancer)
Plain X-Ray and CT scan L4/5.
Note ragged destruction of endplates and adjacent sclerosis L4/5.

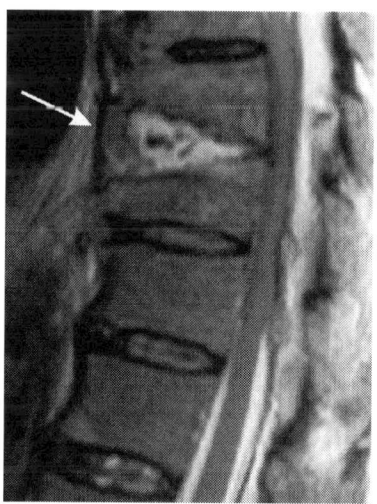

T2 MRI sagittal view thoracic spine with high signal infective discitis.

Discitis

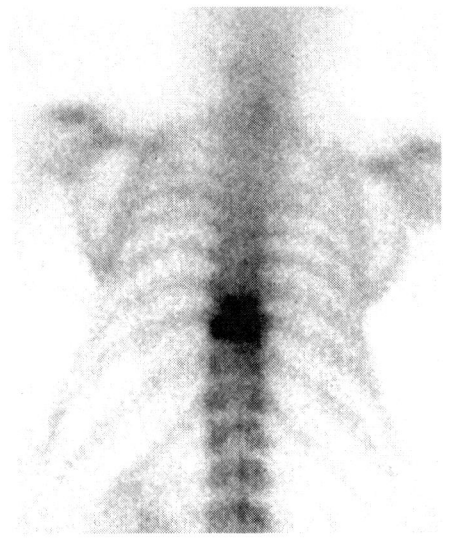

Radio-isotope bone scan: T9/10 discitis (black) but could be cancer metastases.

EMBRYOLOGY

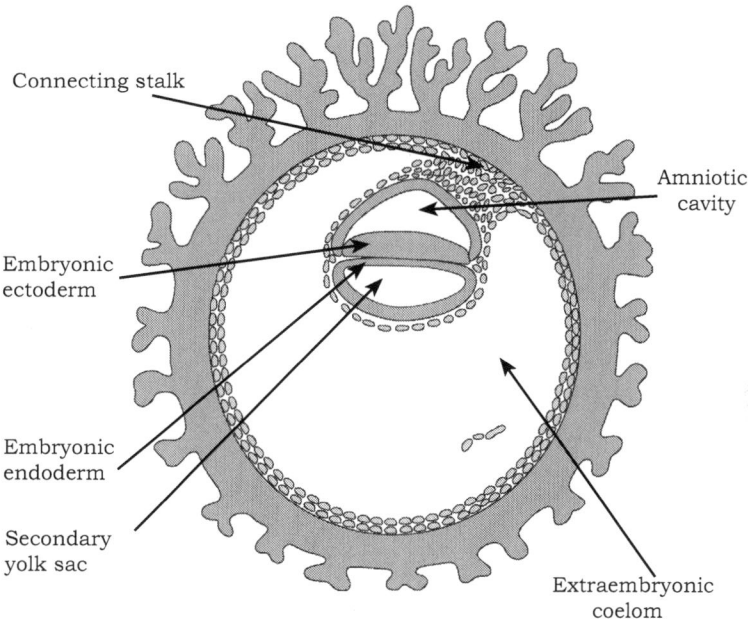

Fig 1 **Two weeks** post fertilization: multicellular blastocyst embeds in uterine wall.

Contains adjoining amniotic sac and yolk sac. Where these sacs meet, they form a cellular two-layered disc.

The **amniotic** sac layer will become the **ectoderm** from which will develop most of the **neural** tissue of the spine.

The **yolk** sac layer will become the **endoderm** producing the notochord which will in turn produce the **nucleus** of the intervertebral discs.

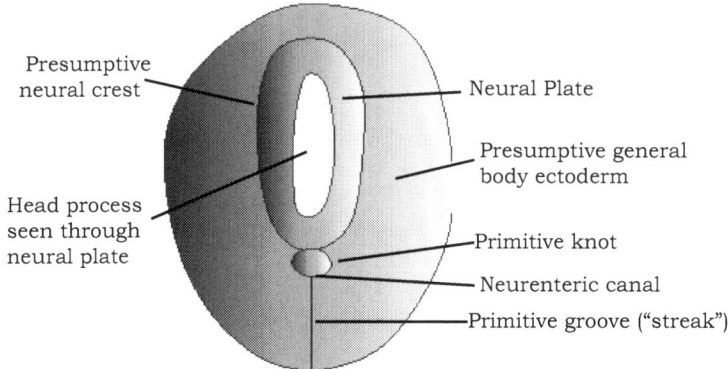

Fig 2 Two weeks post fertilization: plan view of "disc" as if looking down from within amniotic sac. There is a centreline or midline ("**primitive streak**") depicted as if the eventual head (cranial) end of the foetus is North and the eventual tail (caudal) end is South. All the subsequent development of the spine takes place along and around this streak.

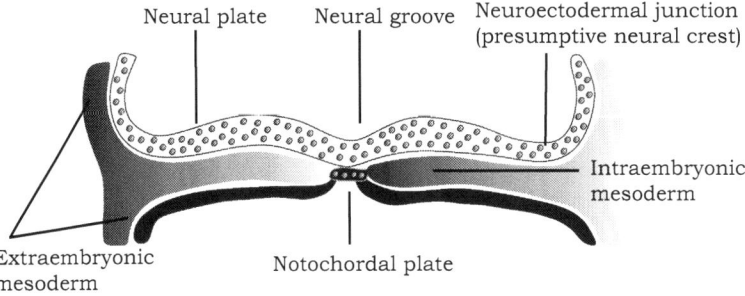

Fig 3 Two to four weeks post fertilization: the two layers become separated (except in the midline) by an invading third layer of **mesoderm**, part of which will produce the **bony vertebral column**.

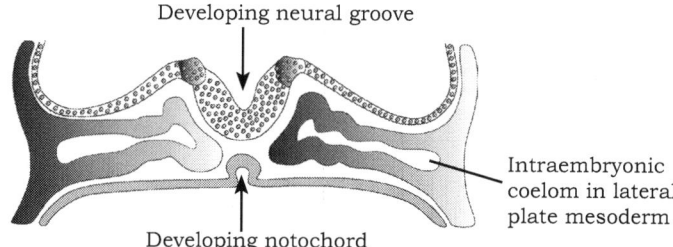

Fig 4 The **ectoderm** starts to heap up on either side of the fixed neural groove, forming peaks which move towards each other.
The **mesoderm** thickens up on either side of the neural groove.
The **endoderm** invaginates upwards in the centreline for the developing notochord.

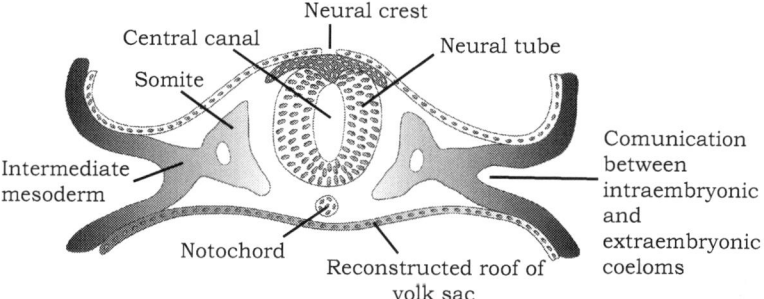

Fig 5 The **ectodermal** peaks meet in the midline dorsally creating the **neural tube** around a central canal. The cells at the joining point form the neural crest, which will eventually develop into the dorsal root ganglia. This sealing up of the neural tube begins near the cranial end of the neural groove and progresses simultaneously cranially and caudally. *If this process is incomplete, the result will be a congenital defect in the form of myelomeningocoele (caudal) or encephalocoele (cranial).* The neural tube will produce the spinal cord and segmental peripheral nerves.
The **mesoderm** develops wedge-shaped thickenings adjacent to the neural tube. At this stage the mesoderm begins to divide up into segments ("**somites**") transversely (see also Fig 7).
The **notochord** has separated from the **endoderm**, which closes over and heals the invagination.

Embryology

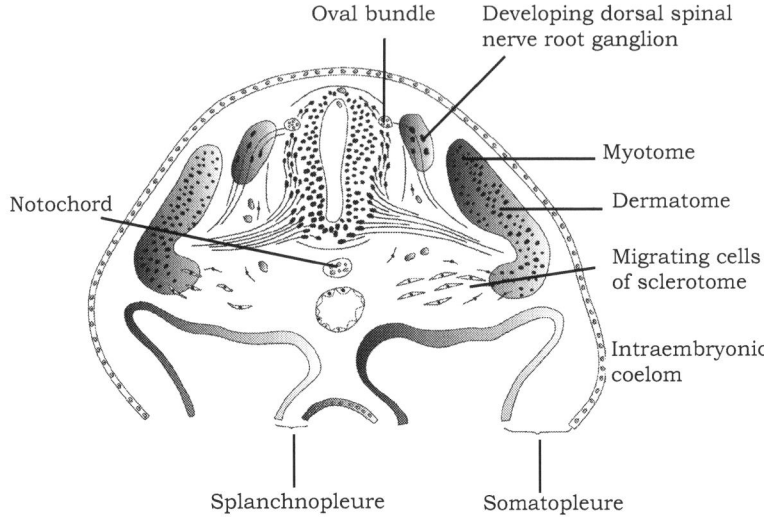

Fig 6 The **neural tube** continues to differentiate, producing the beginnings of segmental nerves and their dorsal root ganglia.
The **mesoderm** differentiates into myotome (muscle), dermatome (skin) and sclerotome (bone).
The **notochord** serves as a focus for **sclerotomal** cells (eventual vertebrae) to cluster around it throughout its length, and in the form of somites.

The neural tube development should be complete by four weeks after fertilization. If closure is incomplete, the scene may set for a varying degree of spina bifida, very likely even before the mother is aware that she is pregnant.

Embryology

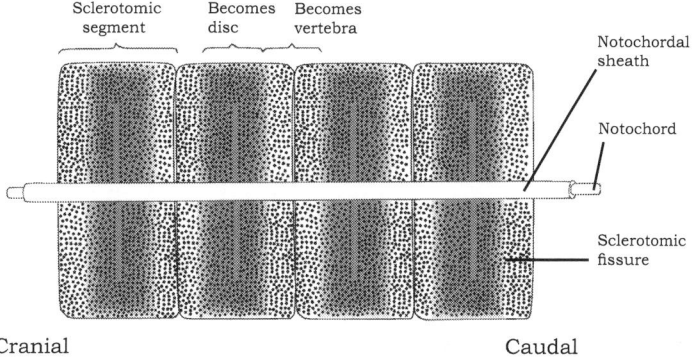

Fig 7   The **vertebrae** form from the adjacent halves of two somites. The **nucleus pulposus** of the intervertebral disc is formed from a segment of the notochord which persists where the somites divide. This division of the somites to form vertebrae is called "resegmentation" and is the focus of controversy among embryologists as to how it comes about. The **anulus fibrosus** (tough outer rim) of the intervertebral disc develops from the rim of each somite.

If somite/vertebra development is defective on one side, this may result in a congenital hemivertebra (wedged from one side to the other) and a resulting scoliosis. If the resegmentation is faulty on one side, the result may be a unilateral unsegmented bar and again, a congenital scoliosis. A combination of wedge vertebrae and an unsegmented bar in the same area of the spine, will produce a severe congenital scoliosis.

EMERGENCIES

There are only two surgical emergencies in spinal disorders practise:

1. CAUDA EQUINA compression [see under]
2. EPIDURAL ABSCESS [see under]

Spinal injury or trauma does not represent a surgical emergency, unless there is a clear deterioration in neurology during the first hours or days after injury. That deterioration may be the result of an enlarging haematoma; surgical evacuation may be useful. Spinal injury may present a treatment emergency in the form of splintage, and the need for catheterisation. No bony injury requires emergency surgery, and no amount of emergency surgery will of itself restore a damaged spinal cord. (See also TRAUMA).

EPIDURAL ABSCESS

One of only two emergencies in spinal disorders. (The other is CAUDA EQUINA SYNDROME, usually the result of a large lumbar central disc prolapse).
- Rare condition.
- Early diagnosis difficult. Paralysis is a common early development.
- Abscess forms at any level in the spinal canal, at any age.
- Staphylococcus aureus, increasingly MRSA. Occasional streptococcus.
- Source is a cryptic septic focus elsewhere in the body: skin, tooth/gums, otitis media.
- Predisposing: diabetes, frequent unsterile venepuncture, trauma, previous spinal surgery, epidural anaesthesia.
- Diagnosis: on suspicion – severe back/neck pain; fever; rigors; high white cell count; high ESR/CRP.
- Emergency MRI for confirmation.
- Treatment: intravenous antibiotics, preferably by central **(picc)** line, flucloxacillin 2gm 6-hourly slow IV, adding vancomycin or linezolid in MRSA; emergency decompression by laminotomy and antibiotic lavage. For very rare multiloculate pan-epidural abscess, use infant feeding catheters to lavage and break loculi distant from laminotomy.

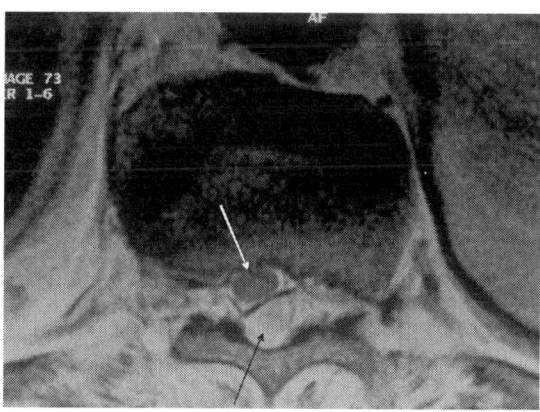

Axial MRI Pyogenic discitis thoracic spine with epidural abscess (white arrow). Spinal cord (black arrow). Paraplegic within hours of start of symptoms.

Epidural Abscess

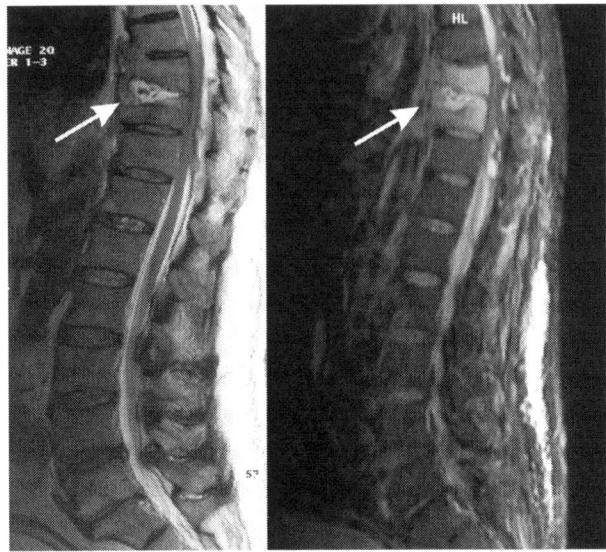

Pyogenic discitis T9/10 MRI T2 on left; fat suppression on right: oedema/pus in adjacent vertebrae.

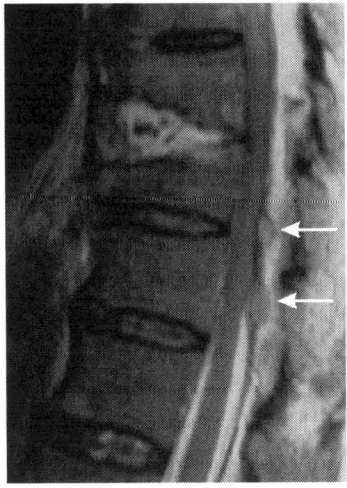

Epidural abscesses, arrowed. Paraplegic on arrival; was ambulant previous day.

EPONYMS [G. *eponymos* = named after]

Apart from all the very similar and confusing Greek terms tormenting the newcomer to Spinal Disorders, there are many eponyms which unnecessarily preserve the aura of mysticism in this discipline.

The best solution would be to abandon the use of eponyms wherever possible, and the author would encourage this strategy. That may sound cruel to the memory of the great men, women and places of medical science, but there are two additional good reasons for moving away from eponyms: there is frequently great disparity between clinicians in the interpretation of the eponymous sign, (or test, angle, instrument, anatomy, pathology, disease, procedure, prosthesis); and there are too many historical aberrations where the name was incorrectly ascribed to a person or place.

Eponyms considered unavoidable in daily use will be so designated in brackets. The author assumes responsibility for any perceived travesties through omission or commission.

Adamkiewicz artery (adam-key-ay-vitch). Medullary feeder artery, vital for spinal cord survival mid-thoracic. Inadvertent ligation during anterior dissection in scoliosis surgery thought to be cause of paralysis. Albert Adamkiewicz 1850-1921, Polish pathologist.

Adams test. Rib hump of scoliosis revealed in forward-bending child, viewed from behind. William Adams 1820-1900, London orthopaedic surgeon, described test in 1864. *Fairbank J. Historical perspective: William Adams, the forward bending test, and the spine of Gideon Algernon Mantell. Spine 29:1953-5, 2004. Rang M. The Story of Orthopaedics. p.153, WB Saunders, 2000.*

Babinski [unavoidable] sign. Extension of big toe and perhaps others, on stimulating sole of foot. Indicates upper motor neurone problem (brain and/or spinal cord). Be afraid, but don't show it. Joseph Babinski 1857-1932, French neurologist.

Batson plexus. Spinal canal dense network of epidural veins draining vertebrae, thought to be passage for spread of spinal infections. Oscar Batson 1894-1979, American otolaryngologist.

Eponyms

Boston brace. Polythene body jacket shaped to counter the deformities of scoliosis but without the need for a neck ring typical of a Milwaukee brace.

Bragard sign. Forced dorsiflexion at the ankle with lower limb raised short of sciatic pain production, looking for reproduction of sciatic pain in suspected lumbar/sacral nerve root compression. Karl Bragard 1890-1973, German orthopaedic surgeon. Attributed also to Polish neurologist J. Fajersztajn, and to Maurice Roch, Austrian (Swiss?) physician. Attribution to Bragard is disputed. *Karbowski K. History of the discovery of the Lasegue phenomenon and its variants. Schweiz Med Wochenschr. 114:992-5, 1984.* (See also **Lasegue**).

Brown-Sequard syndrome. Is unilateral spinal cord lesion. Ipsilateral loss of proprioception and power; contralateral loss of pain, temperature, and light touch sensations. Charles Brown-Sequard 1817-94, French neurologist.

Buck fusion. Operation for low lumbar spondylolysis, placing screws across the fracture, plus bone graft. John Edward Buck 1915-2006, British orthopaedic surgeon. *J Bone Joint Surg 52-B: 432-7, 1970.*

Capener gouge. Characteristic crank in the shank. Also, costotransversectomy approach for thoracic spine TB. Norman Capener, 1898-1975 orthopaedic surgeon, Exeter, UK.

Chance fracture. Horizontal split of vertebral body passing through pedicles and spinous process, thoracic or lumbar, associated with violent distraction force.
GQ Chance, 20th century British radiologist, described in 1948.

Cloward procedure and instruments, for anterior fusions, cervical and lumbar spine. Ralph Bingham Cloward 1908-2000, neurosurgeon, US and Hawaii. Also developed and popularised the posterior lumbar interbody fusion – PLIF, 1943.

Cobb [unavoidable] angle, measured on postero-anterior plain radiograph, indicating severity of scoliosis deformity. Also: elevators for posterior surgical exposure.
John Robert Cobb 1903-67, orthopaedic surgeon, New York, famously said to have declared, "You don't have to be crazy to do scoliosis but it sure helps". Example of mis-attribution:

Cobb states clearly in his classic Instructional Course Lecture of 1948 that he learned the angle measuring technique from Dr Robert **Lippman** in 1935. *Cobb JR: Outline for the Study of Scoliosis. Instructional Course Lectures vol 5. The American Academy of Orthopaedic Surgeons. Ann Arbor, MI, JW Edwards 1948.*

Duchenne [unavoidable] muscular dystrophy. Most common childhood muscular dystrophy; X-linked inheritance affecting males and resulting in death in late adolescence. Guillaume Duchenne 1806-75, French neurologist.

Ehlers-Danlos [unavoidable] autosomal dominant inheritable connective tissue disorders affecting collagen integrity. Generalised hyperelasticity and fragility of skin; joint hypermobility; scoliosis. Edward L. Ehlers 1863-1937, Danish dermatologist. Henri A. Danlos 1844-1912, French dermatologist.

Ewing [unavoidable] tumour, malignant sarcoma of bone, described 1921. James Ewing 1866-1943, U.S. pathologist.

Forestier disease or DISH (diffuse idiopathic skeletal hyperostosis). Condition mainly of lumbar spine, frequently asymptomatic, characterised by dramatically large anterior vertebral body margin osteophytes at several successive levels, discovered incidentally. May indeed be painful. Usually treated by rheumatologists. No surgery necessary. Jacques Forestier (died 1978?) French rheumatologist. *Forestier J, Rotes-Querol J. Senile ankylosing hyperostosis of the spine. Ann Rheum Dis 9:321-330, 1950.*

Frankel [unavoidable, possibly the most quoted eponym in all spinal literature] grades of neurological deficit from "A" (total paralysis) to "E" (normal), applied mostly in traumatic spinal cord injury assessment. See under **Trauma Frankel Grades**. Hans Frankel OBE b.1932, Danzig. *Frankel HL et al. The value of postural reduction in the initial management of closed injuries of the spine with paraplegia and tetraplegia. Paraplegia 7: 179-92, 1969.*

Frazier suction tip. Fine single tube, usually metal, for evacuating blood during spinal operations. Charles H Frazier 1870-1936, US surgeon.

Eponyms

Ghon focus or tubercle. Dormant tuberculous lesion in lung, from childhood infection, calcified and visible on chest x-ray. Anton Ghon 1866-1936, Czechoslovakian pathologist.

Harrington [unavoidable] rod and posterior fusion procedure for scoliosis. Dominated scoliosis surgery for 40 years. Paul Randall Harrington 1911-1980, orthopaedic surgeon, Kansas USA.

Heberden nodes. Are enlarged distal interphalangeal joints in constitutional precocious osteo-arthropathy. William Heberden 1710-1801, English physician.

Hoffmann [unavoidable] sign in cervical myelopathy. Flicking volar surface of terminal phalanx of middle finger (say) produces involuntary flexion of terminal phalanges of thumb and index finger. Also: Werdnig-Hoffmann spinal muscular atrophy. Johann Hoffmann 1857-1919, German neurologist.

Horner [unavoidable] syndrome. Ophthalmic ptosis, miosis, anhidrosis, enophthalmos following injury to or disease of cervical sympathetic chain. Johann F Horner 1831-86, Swiss ophthalmologist.

Kerrison rongeur. Only one of several designs for angled upcutters. Philip D Kerrison 1861-1944, American ENT surgeon, designed instrument as a mastoid rongeur. Also named Ferris-Smith rongeur in some catalogues.

King classification of thoracic idiopathic scoliosis. Guide to segmental levels to be included in fusion to minimise postoperative loss of correction. Although developed in Harrington rod era, still useful. King merely first author of this important paper.
King H, Moe J, Bradford M, Winter R. The selection of fusion levels in thoracic idiopathic scoliosis. J Bone Joint Surg 65-A:1302-13, 1983. **p. 137.**

Klippel-Feil syndrome. Inherited autosomal dominant congenital failure of segmentation of cervical vertebrae. Maurice Klippel 1858-1942, French neurologist. Andre Feil, contemporary of Klippel, French physician.

Lasegue sign: degree to which straight leg raising (SLR) is limited by pain in sciatic distribution in suspected lumbar/sacral nerve root compression. Major disparities of performance and attribution.

Described in 1881 thesis by J-J Forst, student of Lasegue, but attributed by Forst to Lasegue. Both Lasegue and Forst believed the restriction in SLR to be the result of thigh muscle contraction. De Beurmann (1884) concluded that the test was positive because of sciatic nerve stretch. **Lazarevic (1884) likewise, in German, but had published originally in Serbo-Croat in 1880, thus most deserving of the eponym.** Fajersztajn (1901) described the crossed SLR attributable to a large central disc prolapse. Avoid Lasegue eponym at all costs in polite company. Probably the most misinterpreted sign/test in all of orthopaedics. Always ask the patient where the pain is, before you mistakenly record a positive test when the pain limiting the SLR is actually felt in the back. Ernest Lasegue 1816-83, French physician.
Woodhall B, Hayes GJ. *The well-leg-raising test of Fajersztajn in the diagnosis of ruptured intervertebral disc.* J Bone Joint Surg 32-A:786-92, 1950.
Dyck P. *Lumbar nerve root: the enigmatic eponyms.* Spine 9:3-6, 1984.

Lhermitte sign. Sensation of electric shock down spine and into lower limbs on neck flexion, suggestive of cervical cord compression. Jacques Jean Lhermitte 1877 -1959, French neurologist and neuropsychiatrist.

Luschka joints. Small upturned lateral extensions of cervical vertebrae, known also as uncovertebral joints. Hubert Luschka 1820-75, German anatomist. Name attached to many different anatomical structures.

Mackiewicz sign (mats-key-ay-vitch). Femoral nerve stretch test. Eponym routinely used in Poland. Sign recently ascribed to Wasserman (his 1918 paper) but Ignacy Mackiewicz died in 1917. Attributed also to Fajersztajn 1901 and Dyck 1976.
Dyck P. *Lumbar nerve root: the enigmatic eponyms.* Spine 9:3-6, 1984.
Dyck P. *The femoral nerve traction test with lumbar disc protrusion.* Surg Neurol 6:163-6, 1976.

Marfan [unavoidable] syndrome. Inherited autosomal dominant disorder of connective tissue, single gene defect affecting fibrillin1, associated with scoliosis, lens dislocation, and aortic dissecting aneurysm, arachnodactyly, joint laxity, high-arched palate. Antoine Bernard-Jean Marfan 1858-1942, French paediatrician.

Eponyms

Mehta [unavoidable] angle. Difference in angles subtended by ribs at apex of spinal curvature, between left and right sides, in early onset scoliosis. Angle difference <20^0 suggests resolving type (vs progressive type). Min Mehta (b. 1926 Bombay) orthopaedic surgeon, London. President, British Scoliosis Society, 1989-91. Herself a scoliosis sufferer, was major influence in returning surgeons' attention to rib hump and early onset scoliosis.

Meyerding [unavoidable] retractor. Spike-and-blade design for posterior exposure of one side of lumbar spine. Also: grades of overlap (**spondylolisthesis**) of one lumbar vertebra slipped forwards on one below, measured in quarters I to IV. Henry William Meyerding 1884-1969, Minnesota, USA, orthopaedic surgeon.
Wright IP. Who was Meyerding? Spine 28: 733-5, 2003.

Milwaukee brace for the non-surgical management of mild and supple idiopathic scoliosis deformity. Principle = firm pelvic girdle supporting rigid metal uprights to which in turn are attached straps which compress the rib hump, finally conecting to a neck ring. Used first in 1946 by Blount and Schmidt for poliomyelitis. Unsightly and cumbersome. Compliance poor and effectiveness uncertain. Variation of brace used by Bigg in 1882.
Bigg RH. Spinal Curvature, London, Churchill, 1882.
Blount WP, Schmidt AC, Keever ED, Leonard ET. Milwaukee brace in the operative treatment of scoliosis. J Bone Joint Surg 40A:511-25, 1958.

Modic types (mow-ditch). MRI bone marrow shading combinations of bright and dark ("1" and "2") in **spondylosis.** Applied also to infection, **metastasis**. Michael T. Modic, radiologist, USA. See Table: MRI VERTEBRAL MARROW SIGNAL CHANGE. *Modic T, Steinberg P, Ross J, Masaryk T, Carter J. Degenerative disk disease: assessment of changes in vertebral body marrow with MR imaging. Radiology 166:193-9, 1988.*

Oswestry Disability Index (ODI). Developed in 1976 at the Robert Jones and Agnes Hunt Orthopaedic Hospital, Oswestry, Shropshire, by Stephen Eisenstein and Judith Couper at the behest of John O'Brien, for measuring the effect of back pain on daily life activities. Now international and the most quoted outcome score in spinal disorders.

Pancoast [unavoidable] tumour. Lung tumour found high in the apex in patients presenting with upper limb pain and weakness. Every such patient should have a chest x-ray. Henry Pancoast 1875-1939, radiologist USA, described in 1924.

Pennybacker surgical instrument (dissector and elevator). Eponym preferred by neurosurgeons; similar instrument named after Watson-Cheyne by orthopaedic surgeons. Joseph Buford Pennybacker 1907-1983, Professor of Neurosurgery, Oxford.

Perdriolle measurement: of degrees of rotation about the vertical axis, of the apical vertebra in scoliosis, on plain AP radiograph. Rene Perdriolle, contemporary French orthopaedic surgeon.
Perdriolle R, Vidal J. Thoracic idiopathic scoliosis curve evolution and prognosis. Spine 10: 785-91, 1985.

Philadelphia cervical collar/brace.

Pott's disease. Tuberculosis of the spine. Sir Percivall Pott 1714-88, English surgeon.

Prader-Labhart-Willi syndrome. Polyphagia, obesity, short stature, mental retardation, hypotonia, scoliosis; inherited congenital small deletion on paternal chromosome 15. Andrea Prader, Swiss physician; Heinrich Willi, Swiss paediatrician, 1919. (No information on Labhart). *Zellweger H, Schneider HJ. Syndrome of hypotonia-hypomentia-hypogonadism: obesity (HHHO) or Prader-Willi syndrome. Am J Dis Child 115:588-98, 1968.*

Rideau surgical "window" in Duchenne muscular dystrophy. Plateau of respiratory function described by Yves Rideau, French physician, as appropriate opportunity for spinal stabilisation operation.
Rideau Y et al. Respiratory function in the muscular dystrophies. Muscle Nerve 4:155-64, 1981.

Risser [unavoidable] sign. Crude but useful measure of stage of bone maturity in scoliosis children, according to the progress medially of the ossification of the iliac apophysis. Also: frame for application of scoliosis corrective casts; and cast with hinges and turnbuckles for scoliosis correction. Joseph Risser 1892-1982, orthopaedic surgeon, New York. Contemporary of John **Cobb**.
Risser J C. The iliac apophysis: an invauable sign in the management of scoliosis. Orthop Relat res, 11:111-9, 1968.

Eponyms

Romanus lesion. Squared-off appearance of vertebrae in ankylosing spondylitis on lateral plain x-ray; result of inflammatory enthesitis. *Romanus R, Yden S. Destructive and ossifying changes in rheumatoid ankylosing spondylitis. Acta Orthop Scand 22,88-99, 1952.*

Romberg sign of loss of proprioception. Standing patient is obviously unsteady when closing eyes. Moritz H Romberg 1798-1873, German physician. "Walking Romberg" more sensitive. *Findlay GF, Balain B, Trivedi JM, Jaffray DC. Does walking change the Romberg sign? Eur Spine 2009, 18:1528.*

Scheuermann disease. Not a disease but a radiological finding of vertebral body anterior wedging, irregular wavy endplates, and indentations into the vertebral endplates of juvenile and adolescent boys (mainly) with visible kyphosis and backpain. Probably familial/genetic. Better to use "juvenile osteochondrosis". Holger Scheuermann 1877-1960, Danish surgeon. Described 1920.

Schmorl nodes. Part of findings in Scheuermann's juvenile osteochondrosis: domed indentations of intervertebral disc into vertebral endplates . Possibly a pain source. Possibly traumatic. Christian Georg Schmorl 1861-1932, German pathologist. Described nodes 1927.

Schöber [unavoidable] test. In ankylosing spondylitis: measure of lumbar spine stiffness. In erect patient, mark point 10 cms above dimples of Venus and 5 cms below. With maximum forward bending, distance between points should increase minimum 5 cms in normal subjects. Less in ankylosing spondylitis. *Schöber P. The lumbar vertebral column and backache. Münch med Wschr 84:336, 1937.*

Schroeder forceps. Sharp pointed pincer type forceps, similar to vulsellum forceps. Useful for gripping adjacent spinous processes during posterior spinal surgery to identify segmental levels or to assess fusion. Karl LE Schroeder 1838-87, German gynaecologist.

Scott wiring and grafting repair of spondylolysis. Wire technique has appearance on x-ray of outline of a butterfly. *Nicoll RO, Scott JH. Lytic spondylolysis. Repair by wiring. Spine 11:1027-30, 1986.*

Smith-Petersen opening wedge spinal osteotomy for ankylosing spondylitis. Also: tri-flanged nail for fixation of fractured neck of femur. Marius N Smith-Petersen, US surgeon, 1886-1953.

Spurling [unavoidable] test. Provocation for cervical nerve root compression. Lateral flexion with chin elevation provokes ipsilateral upper limb pain and paraesthesiae. Roy Glenwood Spurling, US neurologist 1894-1968; had to care for the tetraplegic General George Patton, early post WWII at US base in Luxembourg.

Tanner & Whitehouse. Atlas of radiographs of stages of maturation of bones of wrist and hand for comparison with those of scoliosis patients, in order to judge likelihood of curve progression. *Tanner JM. Assessment of skeletal maturity and prediction of adult height (TW3 method). 3rd ed. London: WB Saunders; 2001.*

Tarlov cyst. Perineural ballooning of nerve root sleeve of one or more roots of cauda equina, containing CSF. May cause alarming erosion of sacrum. Incidental finding on radiculography or MRI. Considered asymptomatic but controversy persists. Attempts at surgical treatment fraught with complications. Isadore Max Tarlov, US surgeon 1905-1970.

Tokuhashi score. Numerical values applied to a patient with metastatic disease of spine to predict longevity and therefore choice of radical or conservative surgery (see TUMOUR METASTASIS). Yasuaki Tokuhashi, orthopaedic surgeon, Japan. *Tokuhashi Y, Matsuzaki H, Toriyama S, Kawano H, Ohsaka S. Scoring system for the preoperative evaluation of metastatic spine tumor prognosis. Spine 25:1110-3, 1990.*

Trendelenburg gait and test for weak hip joint abductors in advanced hip arthritis: "the sound side sags". Friedrich Trendelenburg 1844-1924, German surgeon.

Waddell signs. Inappropriate and exaggerated responses to 5 gentle manoeuvres, suggesting psychosocial problems or blatant malingering, sometimes over-interpreted by zealous clinicians. Gordon Waddell, contemporary orthopaedic surgeon, Glasgow.
Waddell G, McCulloch J, Kummel E, Venner R. Non-organic physical signs in low-back pain. Spine 5:117-25, 1980.

Eponyms

Watson Cheyne surgical instrument. Dissector and elevator similar to Pennybacker (see above). Likely to be transcribed as "watch-and-chain" by uninitiated clerical staff. Sir William Watson Cheyne 1852-1932, Scottish surgeon and bacteriologist; pioneer of antiseptic techniques with Lister; consultant surgeon to Lord Roberts during Boer War in South Africa 1899-1902.

EXAMINATION

1. The style of examination of the spine set out here is not intended to be comprehensive or exhaustive but sufficiently inclusive to guide the examiner towards a plausible diagnosis within a realistic time limit. Circumstances will demand modifications. Aspirant and practising neurologists will be dissatisfied.

2. Some emphasis is placed on allowing the patient to make most of the moves, retaining control over what is happening. Most patients will be in some pain and therefore apprehensive that the examiner will inflict more pain. Confidence in the examiner and in subsequent procedures may be lost if that apprehension is confirmed.

3. Every examination should follow a probing history. **(see HISTORY).** The reality of professional practice reveals frequent occasions when this is simply not possible. Some conditions such as lumbar spinal stenosis are diagnosed almost entirely on history.

4. Every examination should begin with an observation of stance and gait. Deformity, pain and stiffness, muscle wasting, limb length discrepancy, spasticity, may all provide valuable clues to the direction an examination should take.

Trunk list to one side unfortunately is not diagnostic of one condition: it can be seen in both sciatic nerve root compression and in mechanical low back pain, but its presence would indicate a certain severity in either case. A certain type of limp may be more helpful: with an **antalgic** (pain avoidance) gait as in sciatica, the patient spends more time on the painless lower limb. A **Trendelenburg** gait of hip arthritis has the patient leaning markedly over to the normal side in order to heave the limb with weak hip abductors of hip joint, through for the next step. This patient may not have a spine problem at all. A "floppy foot" or dropped foot gait means dorsiflexion weakness at the ankle, possibly the result of L5 root compression by disc prolapse.

Examination

Dermatomes

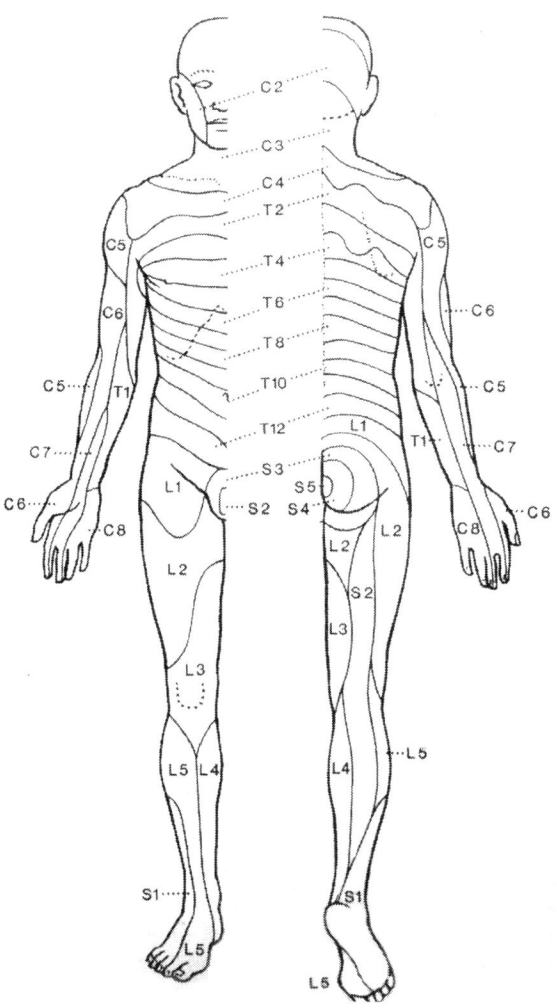

After Keegan JJ (1947) and Garrett FD (1948)

Examination

Cervical spine
- Likely diagnoses: spondylosis = ("wear-and-tear") mainly neck pain and stiffness; radiculopathy (pinched nerve root) = mainly upper limb pain, weakness, paraesthesiae; myelopathy (pinched spinal cord) = upper and/or lower limb weakness with fumbling clumsiness and spastic gait.

- Less likely diagnoses: metastasis; infection; rheumatoid arthritis; ankylosing spondylitis.

- Movement: range and character of: chin on chest, look at ceiling, look left and right. Generalised decrease in range and jerky character with pain, in spondylosis.
- **Spurling**'s test: tip ear onto shoulder then lift chin, left and right. Positive for pinched nerve if severe pain felt down upper limb on side to which head is tipped.
- Sensation: feel volar surface of digits left and right simultaneously asking patient to compare. Numbness and/or paraesthesiae may give clue to pinched nerve. [See Dermatomes]. Patch over deltoid = C5.
- Power: patient to grip examiner's offered index and middle fingers with full strength and then encouraged to resist examiner's attempts to force forearm rotation, flexion, extension.
- Reflexes: looking for reduction as in radiculopathy. Biceps = C5/6; Supinator = C5/6; Triceps = C6/7. Reflex : looking for increase as in myelopathy. Apart from generally brisk reflexes, look also for **Hoffmann**'s sign; little finger lateral escape sign; fine finger movement clumsiness; slow fist-making and release; loss of proprioception and vibration sense including **Romberg** sign; **Babinski** sign; **clonus**.
- Palpate cervical spine and upper thoracic spine posteriorly and posterolateral, looking for marked tenderness of spondylosis or ligamentous strain; trapezius muscle for frequent tender trigger points. Anteriorly to exclude lymphadenopathy.
- Shoulder movements to exclude shoulder girdle problems commonly found together with spondylosis: request hands clasped back of neck; behind back; abduction (sideways lift) of straight upper limbs to touch hands above head.

Examination

Thoracic spine
- Likely diagnoses: common non-specific interscapular pain ("fibrositis", "myalgia"). Also, but less common: metastasis, infection; osteoporotic compression.
- Less likely diagnoses: ankylosing spondylitis; scapulothoracic arthralgia.
- Palpate midline ligaments and posterior musculature especially medial border scapula, for trigger points.
- Percuss spinous processes: exquisite tenderness suggests infection or other infiltrative disease such as metastasis. **(David Jaffray, Oswestry).**
- Respiratory excursion should be 5 centimetres plus. Less in ankylosing spondylitis. Tape measure just below breasts: measure at full inspiration and full expiration.

Lumbar spine
- Likely diagnoses: spondylosis or soft tissue strain = back pain with or without referred (overflow) pain to lower limb; root compression = **sciatica**; spondylolysis = back pain; spondylolisthesis = back pain and **sciatica**; stenosis = spinal claudication.

- Less likely diagnoses: metastasis; infection; spinal cord or cauda equina compression.
  General impression undressed (except underwear): obesity, lordosis, kyphosis, scoliosis, scars of previous surgery.
- Erector spinae tension: see and feel in standing patient; common in back pain and cannot be faked.
- See thigh and calf muscles for wasting, front and rear. Trust your trained eye; no need to measure.
- Bending, flexion and extension: range less important than character. Jerky return or hand-climbing up thighs suggests pain of spondylosis. Pain restricting extension suggests facet arthrosis. Lateral flexion and rotation not helpful.
- Recumbent supine with level pelvis: check for limb length discrepancy and foot pulses: claudication with good peripheral circulation = spinal, not arterial.

- Straight-leg raising, unforced and no more than lightly assisted. If restricted by pain, check whether by **sciatica** (pinched nerve) or by back pain. **WRONGLY INTERPRETED MORE FREQUENTLY THAN ANY OTHER TEST IN SPINAL DISORDERS.**
- Variations for confirmation of sciatica are slump test (patient sitting, lower limbs flexed, neck and thoracic spine slumped forwards before lower limb extended); bowstring test and forced ankle dorsiflexion test. **Crossed straight-leg raising test suggests large central disc prolapse threatening sacral nerves which control perineal sphincters for urinary and faecal continence.**
- Reflexes: knee (L3/4); ankle (L5/S1). Reduction or absence suggest relevant root compression. Intact reflexes in presence of sciatica suggest L5 root compression, most likely at L4/5 disc. **Romberg, Babinski, clonus** suggest upper motor neurone (cord or brain lesion). Loss of proprioception and vibration sense would focus attention on cerebellum and dorsal columns.

  Where there is pain with scoliosis, check abdominal reflexes; absence may indicate spinal tumour.
- Sensation: see **dermatome diagram**. Most common reductions are lateral border foot (S1); big toe and dorsum foot (L5); anterior thigh (L3/4). No diagram is absolute: expect variations and overlaps between patients.
- Pin prick sensation retained in patient paralysed with spinal cord injury, is single most important prognosticator for useful motor recovery.
- Power: resist effort in all directions at ankle joint. Reduced plantar flexion & eversion = S1 weakness; reduced dorsiflexion especially distal phalanx big toe = L5 weakness. Resist knee flexion = L3/4. Resist knee extension = L2/3. Psoas test for L1,2,3 nerve roots: patient sitting with knee kept flexed 90^0 and flexing hip joint against resistance.
- Pulses: dorsalis pedis or posterior tibial (behind medial malleolus). Claudication may be arterial as well as spinal, in the same patient!
- Femoral nerve stretch test: recumbent lateral; gentle hyperextension of hip joint with **decubitus** thigh flexed. Anterior thigh pain suggests **femoratica (or femoralgia)**,

Examination

> compression of the L2,3,4 nerve roots which make up the femoral nerve. Extremely unkind to perform test with patient prone.

- Sacroiliac joint tests are probably irrelevant: significant sacroiliac joint pathology or injury is extremely rare. Stress joint, looking for pain, by placing hip joint in **f**lexion, **ab**duction, **e**xternal **r**otation ("faber" test).
- **Waddell** signs: claimed to represent inappropriate manifestations of back pain in patients exhibiting illness behaviour or outright malingering. Debatable in some respects and misrepresented by some clinicians for medico-legal purposes. Suspect excessive adverse back pain responses to: light pressure on top of head; turning pelvis and spine together; light palpation whole spine; straight leg raising test.

Waddell G, McCulloch J, Kummel E, Venner R. Spine 5:117-25, 1980.

FAILED LUMBAR SURGERY
ALGORITHM FOR MANAGEMENT

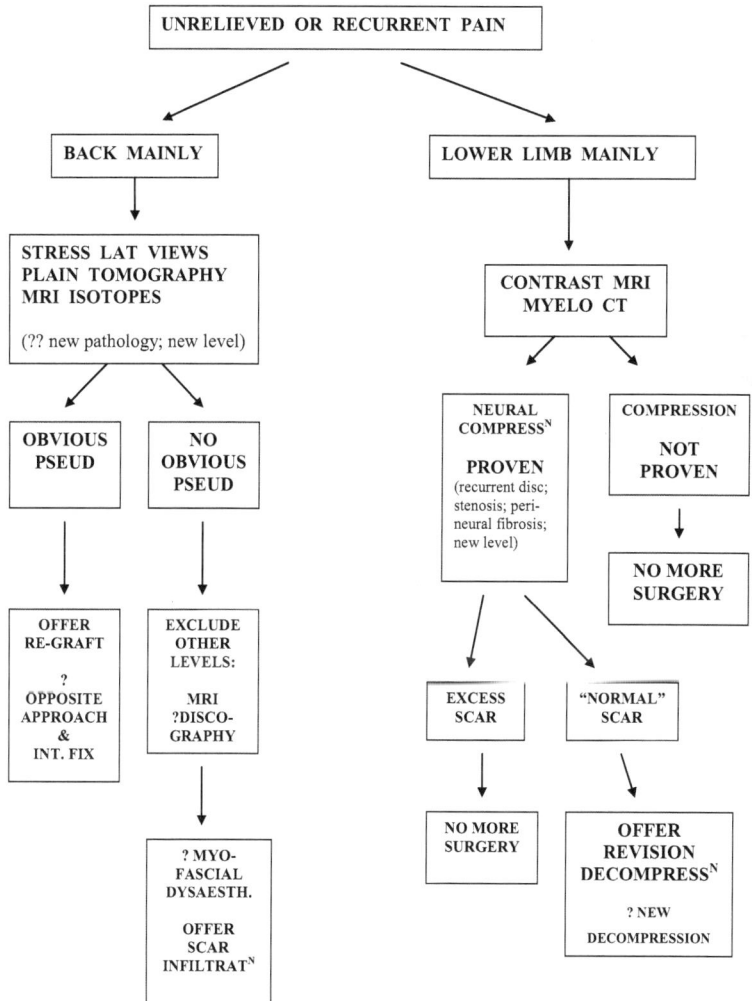

© Stephen Eisenstein.

Eisenstein S. Failed lumbar surgery: Principles of management. J. Bone Joint Surg 1998 80B Supp 2, 149.

FUNCTIONAL RESTORATION

Rehabilitation for daily life activities, aimed at those who are disabled by mechanical back pain, in the absence of significant pathology.

- Combines graduated increase in supervised physical therapy with behavioural techniques of encouragement to achieve physical targets, in spite of pain: Functional Restoration Programme (FRP). "Tough love and PT" modelled on precepts of Mayer and Gatchell.[1] Aim is to demonstrate what is physically possible without causing harm, even if causing hurt. NOT a pain management programme with medications and infiltrations provided by anaesthetists and pain specialists.

- Ideal patient has disability beyond what can be explained by any discoverable pathology ie disordered perception rather than disordered spine. Disabling pain should have been present for at least 3 months. Should be otherwise well enough to undertake exercise; independent for self care; not requiring narcotic medication; not involved in any compensation litigation for spinal problem. Most patients no longer working.

- Suitable also for occasional postoperative patient not achieving full physical potential in spite of technical success.

- FRP ideally lasts 3 weeks, residential Monday to Friday. Patient selection would have begun with outpatient assessment by spine consultant or FRP paramedical specialist, and surgically treatable pathology excluded.

- Selection continues with interview by FRP staff to assess disability, motivation, and to customise programme. Disability is scored by the **Oswestry Disability Index** (ODI) and the Hospital Anxiety and Depression score (HAD) at start of programme, end of programme, and at 6, 12, 18 months.

- <u>Exercises</u> performed in heated pool early in programme, improve confidence. Graduated increases in floor exercises, lifting, and timed walking improve confidence further. Programmes customised to each patient's starting tolerance limits.
 Basic spinal anatomy and physiology explained. Spectres of "crumbling spine" and "wheel chair" dissipated.

Perception of pain eventually diminishes coincident with increased ability.

- <u>Success rate</u> = 72% : return to useful work and daily life activities. Refresher courses of one week sometimes required at 6 month intervals.

[1]*Mayer TG, Gatchell RJ. Functional Restoration for Spinal Disorders: The Sports Medicine Approach. Lea & Febiger, Philadelphia 1988*

GLOSSARY

algorithm Ordered sequence of steps for management of (eg) a health care problem, where each step depends on the outcome of the previous one.
ankylosis Pathological or surgically-intended solid bony continuity across a joint. Stiff fibrous joint restriction occasionally referred to as fibrous ankylosis.
antalgic Refers mostly to a type of gait used to minimise pain, spending least possible time on painful lower limb.
arthralgia Joint pain.
anulus Multilayered fibrous ring-like container of intervertebral disc. (L. anulus = ring).
arthritis Inflammatory or degenerative disease of joints manifesting in pain and stiffness. Appropriate term in presence of proved rheumatoid arthritis, ankylosing spondylitis, gout, psoriasis, and the gut inflammatory arthropathies. Single most abused word in spinal disorders and the cause of unnecessary distress in many patients inappropriately so labelled. Most spinal pain is age related, with relevant radiological changes. Ageing is not a disease. Spondylosis is the correct term for professional use: "wear-and-tear" will do nicely for patients.
arthrodesis General term for any joint fusion operation or established condition, including spinal. Syn: spondylodesis = arthrodesis specifically spinal.
axial Plane or "slice" as in CT or MRI imaging, transversely (plan form) across long axis of body.
biopsy Technique for acquiring tissue sample for histological microscope examination, usually to confirm or refute a presumptive diagnosis of cancer. Most commonly a needle biopsy: tissue acquired within bore of needle. Refers also to tissue sample itself, depending on context.
bisphosphonates Synthetic pyrophosphates, inhibit osteoclast resorption of bone, widely used in treatment of osteoporosis.
calcitonin Peptide hormone, increases deposition of calcium and phosphate in bone, produced by parathyroid and thyroid glands.
cauda equina Includes all the spinal nerves contained within the spinal canal below the level of termination of the spinal cord, generally L1 - L2. "Syndrome" implies varying degrees of lower limb weakness/paralysis with loss of sensation, including perineal sensation, with loss of urinary and/or anal sphincter control. Most common cause is large lumbar disc prolapse.
L. horse tail.
caudal Further down the spine.

Glossary

chylothorax Intrapleural collection of chyle, usually result of injury to thoracic duct during surgery to expose anterior thoracic spine.

claudication Pain in lower limbs on walking. Vascular as in arterial obstructive disease, or Spinal as in spinal stenosis. One patient may manifest both conditions. L. *claudicatio* to limp.

clonus Abnormal repetition of spastic contraction of a lower limb muscle group in response to single sudden imposed stretch. Usually tested at ankle and knee. Indicates upper motor neurone (brain or spinal cord) pathology. G. *klonos* tumult.

coronal Plane or "slice" of anatomy extending left-right ie from side to side, parallel to long axis of body.

costoplasty Excision of sections from a series of ribs. Now part of scoliosis surgery, aimed specifically at correcting unsightly rib hump. *Barrett D, MacLean J, Bettany J, Ransford A, Edgar M. Costoplasty in adolescent idiopathic scoliosis. Objective results in 55 patients. J Bone Joint Surg 75-B:881-5, 1993.*

cranial Further up the spine.

decubitus Surface of patient in contact with bed or operating table eg "left lateral decubitus" = left side down. L. *decumbo* to lie down.

dermatome Ribbon-like area of sensation in skin, served by a single segmental nerve and labelled accordingly. Many "authoritative" versions, differing in matters of detail: Foerster, Fender, Brain, Keegan & Garrett.

diastematomyelia Spinal cord midline split associated with bone or cartilage septum in the split. Septum may damage cord in excessive surgical correction of congenital scoliosis.
G. *diastema* interval; *myelon* marrow.

dysautonomia Abnormal functioning of autonomic nervous system. Early post spinal cord injury; may cause catastrophic hypotension on premature mobilisation.

diplomyelia Duplication of spinal cord in diastematomyelia, but may be no more than split spinal cord.

discectomy Surgical removal of portion of intervertebral disc, usually for disc prolapse with nerve root compression, or in preparation for interbody arthrodesis / disc replacement operations.

enthesitis / enthesopathy Inflammatory erosions where muscles or tendons insert into bone, associated with ossification, especially in vertebrae in ankylosing spondylitis.

femoratica / femoralgia Femoral nerve pain and paraesthesiae (anterior thigh), as distinguished from sciatica. Distinguish also from meralgia paraesthetica.

gibbus Acute angled dorsally-directed deformity of thoracic

spine associated with tuberculosis, trauma, metastasis, congenital deformity. Contrast with smoother deformity of kyphosis.
grade A measure of the severity of cancer according to histological features. Tissue sample usually acquired by biopsy.
idiopathic Cause unknown.
ileus Paralysis of bowel, temporary, especially after transabdominal approach to lumbar spine.
kyphectomy Surgical excision of apex of gibbus or kyphos as in tuberculosis or spina bifida, usually combined with fusion and fixation of the remaining free ends of the spine.
kyphos Used interchangeably with "gibbus".
kyphosis Deformity of spine, usually thoracic, in the form of excessive dorsal prominence but less acute-angled than kyphos or gibbus. In thoracic spine, normal kyphosis generally accepted up to 40^0.
kyphoplasty Technique for correcting kyphosis deformity from vertebral wedge compression fractures: balloon inserted through pedicle inflates to restore height, then maintained by injection of acrylic paste. (See also vertebroplasty).
laminectomy Surgical removal of neural arch of vertebra, single side (hemi-laminectomy) or bilateral; as part of exposure of spinal canal. Term incorrectly used to denote operation to excise prolapsed disc causing nerve root compression.
laminotomy Surgical approach to spinal canal *between* laminae, unilateral or bilateral; removing ligamentum flavum and possibly a little of adjacent edges of laminae. Favoured over laminectomy as being less destructive of anatomy. (Syn. fenestration).
meralgia paraesthetica Pain and paraesthesiae anterior and lateral surfaces of thigh from compression of lateral cutaneous nerve of thigh within inguinal ligament. G. *meros* thigh; *algos* pain.
metastasis Focus of cancer distant from origin, frequently in bone especially spine, and frequently in multiple sites.
myelodysplasia Spinal cord developmental abnormality, especially lower cord, associated with variable lower limb paralysis, urinary incontinence and urinary tract infections. Usually associated with spinal dysraphism ie "spina bifida".
myelogram Radiological demonstration of cauda equina following intrathecal injection of radio-opaque contrast medium to exclude or confirm nerve root compression. Now largely replaced by non-invasive MRI.
myelopathy Clinical presentation of spastic paralysis owing to some spinal cord pathology, compression, or trauma.

Glossary

neoplasia Euphemism for cancer. *G Neo plasis* new growth.
nucleus pulposus Gelatinous soft centre of intervertebral disc.
osteomalacia Subnormal quantity of bone per unit volume because of reduced mineralisation of osteoid. Result of disordered absorption or metabolism of vitamin D and calcium: "tea and toast recluse"; or malnutrition especially in children (rickets).
osteopaenia Inclusive term describing subnormal quantity of bone per unit volume, pathological as in osteoporosis and osteomalacia; or physiological as in childhood growth spurts. Risk of vertebral wedge compression fractures in elderly females.
osteoporosis Subnormal quantity of bone per unit volume but where balance between osteoid and mineral is normal. Most commonly in postmenopausal white women.
pannus Inflammatory synovial tissue in rheumatoid joints. Destroys articular cartilage and bone.
paraesthesiae Abnormal sensations associated with nerve irritation or compression and described variously as tingling, prickling, burning, numbness. Common association with sciatica and cervical radiculopathy.
pars interarticularis Narrow bone bridge between ipsilateral articular processes of vertebra. Site of ununited fracture from childhood, usually lumbar. Oblique plain x-ray shows classical "Scotty dog" with dark neck collar at fracture site. (See SPONDYLOLYSIS)
podagra Severe pain, swelling, discolouration of big toe in acute gout.
prolapse Abnormal bulge of intervertebral disc beyond normal confines, and posing threat of neural compression. Classified in terms of increasing severity of bulging: protrusion; extrusion; sequestration.
proprioception A sense of the position of the body and its limbs in space, independant of vision.
pseudarthrosis Literally: false joint. Used to describe gap in spinal fusion graft mass, or gap between fracture ends long after bone healing would have been expected. May be cause of persisting pain after bone transplant surgery, eg failed spinal fusion.
radiculopathy Clinical syndrome of single nerve root ("radicle") compression or irritation: limb pain, paraesthesiae, weakness, diminished sensation, diminished reflexes. Disc prolapse with nerve root compression is most common cause, neck or low back.
radiculogram Radiological demonstration of cauda equina nerve root ("radicle") sleeves following intrathecal injection of radio-opaque contrast medium to exclude or confirm nerve root compression. Most common indication is lower limb pain due to

Glossary

suspected lumbar disc prolapse. Falling into disuse with availability of non-invasive MRI. Term often used interchangeably with myelogram.

Red Flags: Symptoms which suggest the uncommon possibility of some serious underlying pathology eg cancer, infection, inflammatory or metabolic disease, large central disc prolapse, requiring further investigation. These symptoms are: constant pain; night pain; weight loss, loss of appetite, rigors, sweats, fever, swelling of large joints, weakness of limbs, loss of perineal sphincter control.

sagittal Cranio-caudal plane or "slice" of anatomy extending from front to back ie anteroposterior. L. *sagitta* arrow.

sciatica Pain and paraesthesiae in part or whole of lower limb, crudely in distribution of one or more dermatomes of nerve roots comprising sciatic nerve; most frequently result of nerve root compression by disc prolapse in lumbar spine. Difficult to distinguish from "referred" pain spreading into lower limb from severe low back pain, and therefore somewhat overdiagnosed.

scoliosis Curvature of spine in coronal (side-to-side) plane, of various origins, often associated with vertebral rotation about the vertical axis.

spina bifida (see myelodysplasia). Spina bifida occulta is a harmless failure of fusion of the two halves of a neural arch, usually lumbar. Congenital, discovered on a plain x-ray.

spondylitis Inflammatory disease of spine eg rheumatoid; ankylosing; infective. Often used by mistake instead of "spondylosis" when describing degenerative or ageing changes.

spondylodesis Spinal fusion, operation or established condition. Syn: arthrodesis.

spondylolisthesis Shift or translation of one vertebral body on the one next below, in any direction, but most commonly anteriorly. "Spondylo" for short. Most common pathology is disc dehydration or degeneration; and spondylolysis (defect in pars interarticularis).

spondylolysis Ununited fracture of pars interarticularis (narrow bridge between superior and inferior articular processes). Never congenital failure of fusion of ossification centres. Maximum incidence ages 6 to 10 years. Usually found low lumbar spine. Usually asymptomatic until adulthood.

spondyloptosis Situation of vertebra shifted so far forward as to have lost support from vertebra below and tending to slide down anterior to lower vertebra.

spondylosis Single word describing a spinal segment with all the changes of age-related degeneration: loss of disc height/hydration; sclerotic vertebral body end-plates with osteophytosis;

Glossary

facet joint hypertrophy and osteophytosis; intra-osseous vertebral cyst formation; spondylolisthesis. Sometimes mistakenly referred to as "spondylitis".

stage A measure of the extent of spread of a cancer beyond its tissue and organ of origin. A variety of imaging techniques always required for proper staging.

subluxation Abnormal separation of joint surfaces but less than total loss of contact as would describe dislocation. In spinal context, applies to facet joints and interbody joints with disc. Seen in trauma and spondylosis.

syndesmophyte Large vertebral body margin osteophyte, often closely meeting with similar from adjacent vertebra (see DISH and ANKYLOSING SPONDYLITIS).

vertebroplasty Injection of fast-setting acrylic paste into vertebral body via pedicle, in osteoporotic fracture and metastasis, to limit or prevent collapse. (See also kyphoplasty).

HISTORY

General

- "HISTORY" comes after "EXAMINATION" here, because of the alphabet, but in practise, taking a good history always comes before conducting a clinical examination.
- **Age**: Much of the clinical assessment of spinal pain, for instance, has to do with what is compatible with patient's age.
- **Occupation**: Many spinal disorders should allow continued employment in sedentary occupations, but may not be appropriate to the current trend of 12-hour shifts in physically demanding jobs.
- **Family circumstances**: A frail elderly patient living alone without family or caring close neighbours, for instance, will require special consideration for disposal after treatment in hospital.
- **Complaints**: Expect almost all patients to present with pain in spine and/or limbs; stiffness in spine, very often with pain; deformity is least likely but a list to one side often accompanies severe back pain; weakness in one or both lower limbs = unusual = RED FLAG for neural compression. Pain worse at night = RED FLAG for neoplasia.
- **General health, past and present**: Hypertension, diabetes, stroke, asthma, COAD, gut sensitivity, joint replacement, deep vein thrombosis, pulmonary embolus, osteoporosis, smoking and alcohol consumption, may all affect treatment programmes, especially in planning for surgery and the consenting process in terms of complications. Smoking carries a high association with pseudarthrosis after spinal fusion.
- **Red Flags**: Symptoms which suggest the uncommon possibility of some serious underlying pathology eg cancer, infection, inflammatory or metabolic disease, large central disc prolapse, requiring further investigation. These symptoms are: constant pain; night pain; weight loss, loss of appetite, rigors, sweats, fever, swelling of large joints, weakness of limbs, loss of perineal sphincter control.

- **Medication**: A surprising number of back pain patients have never taken standard analgesics. Anti-inflammatory medications are suspected of having an adverse effect on bone grafts in spinal fusion surgery. Anti-coagulant therapy will provide an interesting time during surgery if not known about previously.

Cervical
- Know that vast majority of patients will have spontaneous onset pain and stiffness from benign cervical **spondylosis.**
- Pain and stiffness in neck: duration and severity, and diurnal variation?
- Radiation to upper limbs? Occipital headache?
- Disability: effect on quality of life, sleep, occupation, leisure, driving?
- Treatment to date: have all the non-surgical options been exhausted?
- Injury? Most likely = known "whiplash" in rear-end RTA shunt. Better to change terminology to "neck sprain" until more serious injury discovered.

- *Serious conditions:* Upper limb pain worse than neck pain, with paraesthesiae and perception of weakness = possible cervical root compression. Clumsy fingers, cannot pick up small objects or do up buttons = possible cervical myelopathy. Intractable 24-hours pain, worse at night = suspect metastasis or infection; after injury, suspect fracture/dislocation.
- *Traps:* Upper limb pain = rarely result of Pancoast tumour in lung; all cervical radiculopathies should have chest x-ray before surgery. Hand / forearm pain may be median nerve compression ("carpal tunnel"); order nerve conduction studies.

History

> Thoracic
> - Know that the vast majority of patients will have benign interscapular pain of chronic mild ligamentous strain.
> - Pain between shoulder blades, spontaneous onset? Relieved by recumbency? Aggravated by physical effort, lifting, pushing?
> - Interscapular pain with intense girdle pain = suspect intercostal neuralgia of osteoporotic vertebral compression fracture.
> - *Serious conditions:* Intractable 24-hours pain, worse at night = suspect metastasis or infection; after injury, suspect fracture/dislocation. Pain with spastic gait = myelopathy = cord compression by tumour, infection, disc prolapse, spondylosis, until proved otherwise.
>
> Lumbar
> - Know that the vast majority of patients will have benign mechanical low back pain of lumbar **spondylosis** or soft tissue strain or facet arthrosis.
> - Know that radiation to lower limbs is common and not likely to be root compression <u>if back pain greater than lower limb pain.</u>
> - If lower limb pain much more severe than back pain, and with paraesthesiae = suspect root compression by disc prolapse or root canal stenosis.
> - Mechanical back pain: Greater with effort and relieved by rest = "strain" type. Greater at rest, relieved by movement = "facet arthrosis" type. Of no great importance to distinguish, <u>but don't dismiss pain at rest as sign of malingering.</u>
> - Back pain with lower limb pain only on walking, and distance steadily reducing because of lower limb pain, weakness and paraesthesiae = lumbar stenosis until proven otherwise.
> - The <u>"locked back attack"</u> = very real entity of very sudden onset of crippling low back pain with spasm following a minimal and innocent postural change, producing bed-bound disability for days to weeks. Cause unknown, but long prior history of "strain" type low back pain is common.

IMAGING

There is a lot more to imaging the spine than mere "x-rays". While plain x-rays are important, the newer scanning technologies of Computed Tomography (CT) and Magnetic Resonance Imaging (MRI) have increased our diagnostic capability enormously. Spine specialists of a certain mature age wonder daily how it was possible to practise with any competence before the advent of these facilities. On the other hand, in this brilliant "new age" there is a danger that imaging is being allowed to provide an excuse for surrendering clinical acumen to the history books.

- **Plain x-ray,** reveals general spine structure, but cannot show details of soft tissues such as muscles, ligaments, discs, and nerves. This examination has become controversial because of what is considered to be high radiation exposure, especially for the lumbar spine. The author remains enthusiastic for the ability to achieve these images quickly, for the sake of demonstrating to the patient that (in the vast majority of cases) any visible pathology is likely to represent little more than "wear and tear". Reassurance, where possible, is a major component of treatment, especially in the emotive arena of spinal disorders. Standard views are a front-to-back (AP = anteroposterior); and a side view (lateral) of the section the spine where the trouble seems to be located. The AP is useful for showing any of the common variations of anatomy especially at the lumbosacral junction (and which could lead to miss-counting segments when operating); the state of the pedicles (an absent pedicle could be the first sign of cancer spread from elsewhere); the psoas muscle shadows (absence could be confirmation of tuberculosis); the sacroiliac joints for early signs of inflammatory disease; and curvatures (scoliosis) of all kinds. The lateral view will reveal changes from the normal clean square appearance of the vertebral bodies (osteoporosis, cancer, infection, congenital) and all the signs of spondylosis, spondylolysis, spondylolisthesis.

- **CT scan,** as the name would suggest, produces computer-generated images from multiple x-ray slices generated by an x-ray source which sweeps around the patient's body. These slices of anatomy can be re-formed in any desired plane. Additional software enables the creation of dramatic 3D images. CT scans are useful for excellent bone detail, especially useful in suspected spine fractures, infections, and tumours. Newer MDCT machines (Multiple Detector CT) are extremely quick and the detail is even finer. When needle biopsy is required, CT is the best imaging for guiding the needle accurately. Soft tissues can be made visible so that disc prolapse (for instance) can be diagnosed, but not with the clarity available on MRI. As with plain x-rays, there is concern regarding radiation exposure.

- **MRI (Magnetic Resonance Imaging),** is the major spinal imaging technique used today. It is remarkable for the clarity with which it displays soft tissue anatomy. Even more important, because of its ability to distinguish between fat and fluids, (the so called STIR sequence), it reveals the state of physiology of the spine and any pathological change in the bone and soft tissues. Not only is the detailed anatomy of each disc seen (anulus separate from nucleus), but all degrees of disc dehydration, the earliest sign of spinal ageing. Nerves are well displayed, as are any neural compressions caused by disc prolapse or stenosis. Infections, inflammations, and tumours show up equally well. Software can reproduce images in any desired plane, but bone detail is not as well defined as with CT.

The scanner is a very powerful magnet (there is no ionising radiation). The patient must lie in a narrow metal tube (and this may create a problem for the claustrophobic). The basis of imaging is proton mapping. All the hydrogen atoms in the water molecules are momentarily converted into mini-magnets aligned along a magnetic field. The images are captured from the proton energy dissipation when the hydrogen atoms return to their original location and orientation. At different stages of the process, different shadings of the tissues are achieved ("T1" and "T2" for instance), improving the quality of diagnosis (see Modic classification p.108). The procedure is expensive, but frequently essential to modern diagnosis and treatment. Intravenous injection of a contrast medium (gadolinium) can highlight the difference between inflamed scar tissue, tumours, blood vessels, and normal tissue.

Imaging

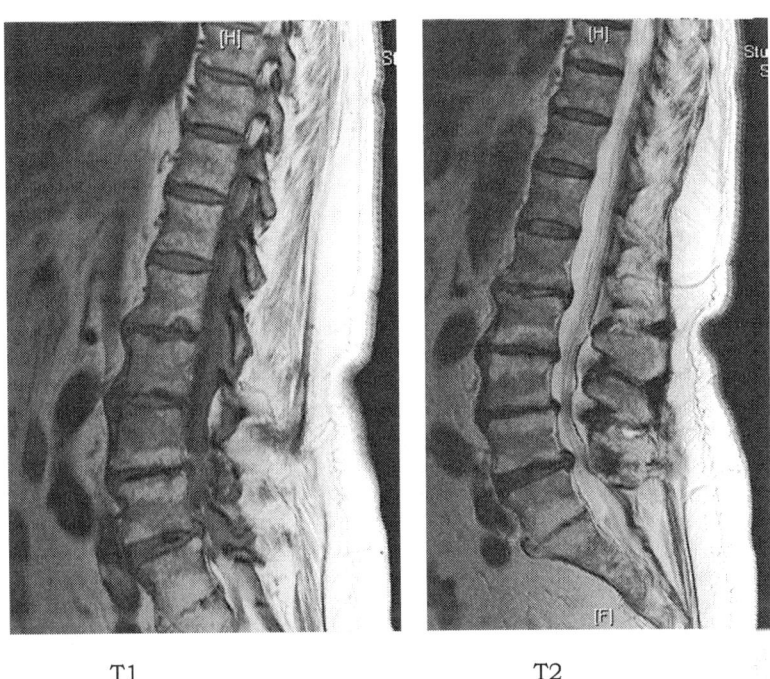

T1 T2

Typical features of spondylosis in middle age. Lumbar spine sagittal view as if patient facing to the left. Note T2 shows up nerves and fluid in spinal canal better than T1.

Imaging

- **Myelography/radiculography,** is the demonstration of the contents of the spinal canal and its neural contents (cord and cauda equina) after the injection of a radio-opaque contrast medium via a lumbar puncture. Prior to the advent of MRI, this was the principal technique of confirming suspected neural compression. It is still much used in the third world where expensive scanners are not available but has been entirely replaced by MRI elsewhere. Its usefulness is limited because the contrast medium cannot flow beyond the termination of the nerve root sleeves and therefore cannot demonstrate far lateral nerve root compressions. The contrast medium frequently causes disabling headache, nausea, and vomiting, for days to weeks. The earliest form of contrast medium was oil-based and potentially toxic to nerves, causing long term neuritis in some patients.

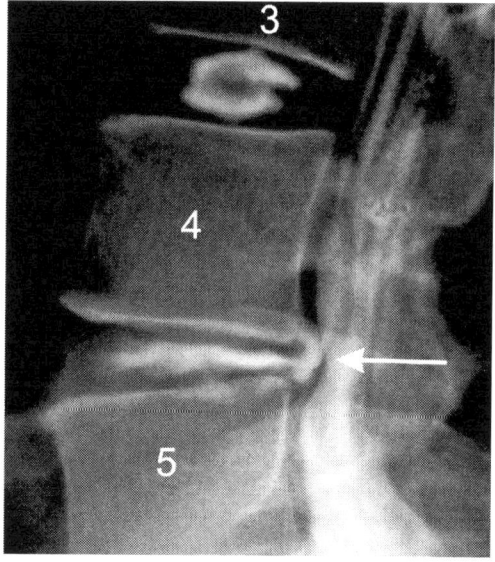

Myelogram of lumbar spine with discography of L3/4 disc (normal) and L4/5 (dehydrated, flattened and protruding onto cauda equina - arrowed). L3/4 discogram is normal because only nucleus can be shown and was painless. L4/5 discogram is abnormal because contrast spreads throughout and typical back pain was reproduced.

- **Discography,** involves the injection of contrast medium into an intervertebral disc under x-ray control, most likely one or more lumbar discs suspected to be sources of pain, and cervical spine discs less frequently. A positive result depends on the contrast medium demonstrating the characteristic morphology of a degenerate disc **PLUS** the experience of typical pain coinciding with the injection. It is possible that the results of spinal fusion surgery for back pain / neck pain were improved by selecting the positive segments for treatment. Unfortunately, the pain from disc injection was so unpleasant that for many patients the memory of that pain overwhelmed any perceived benefit from fusion surgery.

Also, bacterial discitis is a known complication of discography, with significantly disabling consequences. This investigation is now little used, having been superseded by MRI, in spite of the fact that MRI cannot distinguish a painful disc from one that is painless.

- **Facet arthrography,** like discography, was intended to define those facet joints (in the lumbar spine particularly) which reproduced the patient's typical facet arthrosis pain on provocation by the injection of contrast medium into the lower three (usually) joints on one or both sides. Unlike discography, there is no typical radiological appearance of facet joint arthrosis. This investigation has also been abandoned somewhat, following some doubt as to the relevance of the findings to success or failure of spinal fusion surgery for back pain. The technique continues to be used for pain management in some centres, providing the opportunity to inject a combination of local anaesthetic and steroid into the painful facet joints.

- **Radio-isotope** in the form of Technetium^{99} is taken up by bone normally, but markedly where there is increased bone turnover; these areas show up as black spots or smudges. It is most useful in revealing the extent of spread of cancer, not only in the whole spine but in the whole skeleton. Infection and arthritis will also be revealed but these would be incidental findings. The isotope is injected intravenously and the scan is done 3 hours later. The findings in cancer are useful for planning treatment. Caution: primary bone marrow cancer (myeloma) may not show up on isotope scan.

Imaging

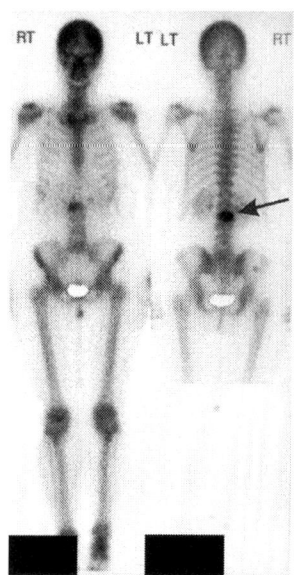

Front and rear views of whole body radio-isotope scan. Normal except for "black spot" (arrowed) of vertebral metastasis at thoraco-lumbar junction.

- **Arteriography** for diagnosis in spinal disorders is rarely required these days. It is used in conjunction with embolisation (the intentional blocking of an artery) to starve a tumour of blood. This technique is of critical importance in preparing a patient for excision of tumours spread to the spine and known to be very vascular. Intra-operative haemorrhage could otherwise be catastrophic. The most notorious such tumour is renal carcinoma in the spine in the adult, and should be embolised 48 hours before surgery to remove a cancerous vertebra.

- **Ultrasound** has little place in adult spinal disorders but will reveal spina bifida in the developing foetus on routine antenatal scanning and congenital spinal abnormalities in the neonate. No radiation is involved nor any injection required; it is therefore very safe. The images are created by capturing the "echo" of high frequency inaudible sound waves returning from tissues of differing density.

INFECTION

1. Bone (vertebrae) = OSTEOMYELITIS [see under]
2. Spinal canal = EPIDURAL ABSCESS [see under]
3. Disc = DISCITIS [see under]
4. Soft tissue = WOUND INFECTION; COMPLICATIONS [see under]

INFLAMMATORY ARTHRITIS

- Represented by a group of loosely related conditions.
- All can cause spinal pain and stiffness but not all patients demonstrate spinal pathology on x-ray.
- Most conditions produce detectable sacro-iliitis and spondylitis.
- Osteoarthritis of the spine is discussed separately (under SPONDYLOSIS) indicating the presumption that this condition has more to do with ageing and degeneration ("wear and tear") than primarily with inflammation.
- The two most important conditions in terms of frequency and spinal pathology, are Ankylosing Spondylitis (AS) and Rheumatoid Arthritis (RA). Consult reference texts (esp. Apley's System of Orthopaedics and Fractures, *Ed.* Solomon L) for the other conditions listed hereunder.

1. Ankylosing Spondylitis [see under ANKYLOSING SPONDYLITIS; SPONDYLITIS]
2. Rheumatoid Arthritis [see under SPONDYLITIS]
3. Reiter's Disease: urethritis, conjunctivitis, uveitis, colitis, dermatitis.
4. Gout: hyperuricaemia, **podagra**, tophi in fingers and toes.

Inflammatory Arthritis

5. Seronegative Polyarthritis
   - Psoriatic arthritis
   - Juvenile chronic arthritis (Still's disease)
   - Systemic Lupus Erythematosis (SLE)

6. Calcium Pyrophosphate Deposition Disease (CPPD): chondrocalcinosis of large joints and intervertebral discs.

7. Polymyalgia Rheumatica: pectoral and pelvic muscle pain in middle-aged women; high ESR.

8. Enteropathic Arthritis
   - Crohn's disease
   - Ulcerative colitis

JARGON and MISNOMERS

"arthritis" Explanation too frequently offered to patients presenting with some musculoskeletal pain, without clinical justification, but in the hope of calming a situation of alarm, and unaware of the greater alarm thereby created.

"fusion" Used to describe a bone transplant operation, ascribing to surgeons the miracles performed by biological processes. Surgeons plant the bone graft; biology makes the fusion (but not always successfully).

"instability" No single word has created more confusion and misapprehension while so devoid of meaning, in the last 30 years of spinal disorders practise. Originally used to explain low back pain, but more sinister use = when excusing a recommendation for spinal fusion surgery. Has different meanings for different disciplines: biomechanics (readings from stress/strain machines); radiology (visible abnormal shift of one vertebra upon another); clinical presentation (pain with movement, relieved by rest). Best abandoned.

"laminectomy" Archaic term for a surgical procedure to excise a prolapsed intervertebral disc causing "sciatica". Laminectomy is not an operation: it is an excessively destructive means of exposing the spinal cord or cauda equina, now little used. Correct term would be "nerve root decompression", and performed through a laminotomy, preserving the midline anatomy as best possible.

"lower leg" The lower limb is divided into the *thigh* (above knee); *leg* (below knee); and *foot* (for sake of completeness). The "lower leg" is not a valid anatomical concept except perhaps in magazines found at the hairdresser. Likewise, the upper limb above the elbow is the arm, and the forearm is below the elbow, not counting the hand.

"referred pain" Meant to explain the concept of pain so intense at point of origin that it tends to flow beyond its rightful anatomical confines. Meaningless by itself; origin unknown. Angina overflowing into left upper limb is a good example; various theoretical neurological explanations eg spinal cord synapses overwhelmed etc. Most common example in spinal disorders is

Jargon and Misnomers

low back pain overflowing into lower limb, groin, testes/labia, in the absence of any neural compression or irritation. Anything wrong with "overflow pain", until the neurological mechanism becomes known?

"sciatica" By custom through the ages, implies lower limb pain, explained on the basis of some lumbosacral nerve root compression or irritation, even in the absence of any evidence to confirm nerve root involvement. Most common cause of root pain is known to be disc prolapse. Numerically, "referred pain" is a far more common cause of lower limb pain than "sciatica" but too many doctors feel their standing is enhanced by calling all lower limb pain "sciatica".

KYPHOSIS [G.humpback]

- "Hunchback" posteriorly protruding deformity, most commonly used to describe the deformity of the thoracic spine in TB or **Scheuermann's** disease or ANKYLOSING SPONDYLITIS, or congenital deformity or the "dowager hump" of osteoporosis.

- Opposite of LORDOSIS.

- Kyphosis usually implies a smooth curve, whatever the severity, whereas **gibbus** describes a sharp deformity such as seen in advanced TB of the thoracic spine, or congenital deformity.

- Kyphoscoliosis describes a combined appearance of kyphosis with lateral curvature of the spine.

- In Scheuermann's disease, modified Milwaukee brace very effective in juveniles. Apply to curves $50°$ to $70°$.

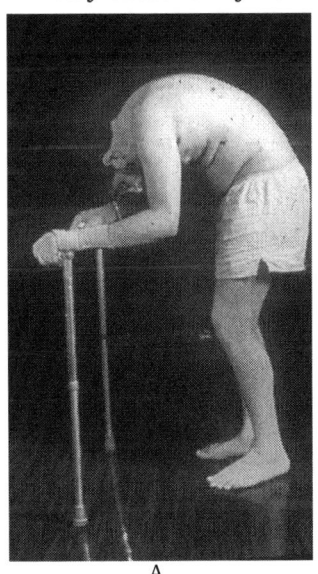 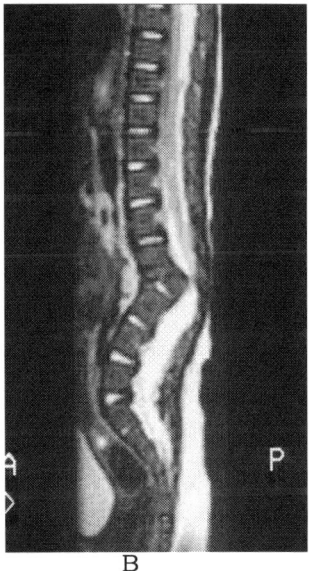

A   B

A: shows smooth but severe kyphosis of anklosing spondylitis.
B: shows sharp gibbus of congenital deformity.

Kyphosis

- Beyond 70°, surgical correction necessary but there is a tendency to high technical complication rate with failure of correction.

- In ankylosing spondylitis, surgical correction of thoracic kyphosis is performed in the lumbar spine by posterior closing wedge osteotomy; correction of the rigid curve in the thoracic spine is associated with a high rate of cord damage and paralysis (See p.17).

Just as there are normal lordosis curves (cervical and lumbar spine), so there is a balancing normal kyphosis in the thoracic spine, up to 40 degrees as measured on a lateral plain film taken in the erect position.

LORDOSIS [G. a bending backward]

- Refers to any forward (anterior) curve of the spine occurring in the **sagittal** plane.

- Opposite of kyphosis.

- Cervical and lumbar spine are normally lordotic. Wide range of normal curvature.

- Hyperlordosis = excessive lordosis, especially as compensation for increased kyphosis in thoracic spine pathology. Common and painful consequence of **Scheuermann** juvenile osteochondrosis.

- Relative lordosis in thoracic spine in idiopathic scoliosis: really a diminished kyphosis.

- Treatment seldom necessary or possible other than treatment of primary pathology eg surgical correction of thoracic kyphosis.

MRI VERTEBRAL MARROW SIGNAL CHANGE

	T1 MRI BONE SHADE	T2 MRI BONE SHADE	MARROW HISTOLOGY
EARLY DISC DEGEN. MODIC 1	DARK	BRIGHT	OEDEMA
LATER DISC DEGEN. MODIC 2	BRIGHT	BRIGHT	FAT
CHRONIC DISC DEGEN. MODIC 3	DARK	DARK	BONE SCLEROSIS FIBROSIS
INFECTION*	DARK	BRIGHT	PUS, OEDEMA, INFLAMMATION
METASTASIS* (EXCEPTION = OSTEOBLASTIC eg PROSTATE)	DARK (DARK)	BRIGHT (DARK)	TUMOUR

* **"T1-2 CHANGER MAY MEAN DANGER"**

Reference: Modic MT, Steinberg PM, Ross JS, Masaryk TJ, Carter JR. Degenerative disk disease: assessment of changes in vertebral body marrow with MR imaging. Radiology: 194:193-9, 1988.

MUSCLE POWER
MEDICAL RESEARCH COUNCIL GRADING

0 = No movement.

1 = Flicker only.

2 = Positive movement but not possible against gravity.

3 = Positive movement against gravity but not against resistance.

4 = Movement against resistance but less than normal.

5 = Normal full strength movement against resistance.

NECK AND UPPER LIMB PAIN

1. Pain in the neck at some stage in life is almost as common as low back pain.
2. Like the rest of back pain, high or low, it is rarely the result of serious disease.
3. Any part of the cervical spine anatomy is capable of transmitting pain sensation.
4. Pain may be sufficiently severe to spread down one or both upper limbs, very much as back pain can spread into the lower limbs, without invoking any nerve root compression.
5. Other areas to which pain may spread: occiput; high thoracic midline; trapezius; supraclavicular and pectoral areas; mandible.
6. Most common radiological finding is cervical spondylosis ("wear and tear" changes of sclerosis, facet joint enlargement, loss of disc height, osteophytosis, **spondylolisthesis**). Do not label "arthritis": patient will perceive imminent crippledom.

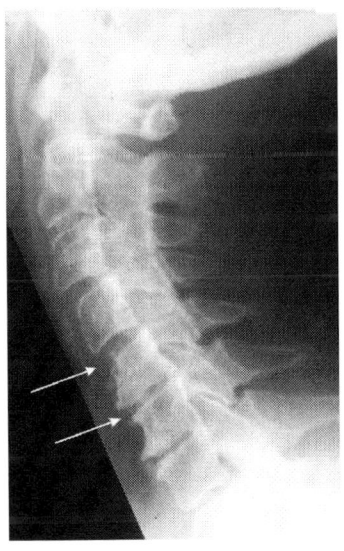

Cervical spine lateral plain x-ray.
Top arrow shows normal disc space C4/5. Bottom arrow shows spondylosis at C5/6 (and C6/7).

Neck and Upper Limb Pain

7. **Where upper limb pain is more intense than neck pain, and associated with paraesthesiae and perceived weakness, suspect neural compression.**
8. Most common cause of neural compression is disc prolapse; then **spondylosis**, especially posterolateral vertebral body marginal osteophytes.

Management – mainly neck pain
- 3-6 weeks = observation; possibly standard analgesics.
- 6-12 weeks = standard analgesics; physiotherapy especially mobilisation; plain x-rays; blood tests FBC, U&E, ESR, RA latex, Uric acid.
- 12 weeks plus, intractable = refer to surgeon.
- Surgeon may (unusually) offer cervical spine fusion, two levels maximum, if MRI confirms no more than two adjacent levels of spondylosis, and if symptoms out of control.
- Significant disease (metastasis, infection, inflammatory disease): treat as indicated for each.
- Chronic, multilevels, unsuitable for surgery: standard analgesics including anti-inflammatories; any combination of gentle manipulative techniques; intermittent soft or hard collar for comfort.

Management – mainly upper limb pain
- 3-6 weeks - standard analgesics; plain x-rays; blood tests.
- 6 weeks plus: refer to surgeon.
- Surgeon may offer anterior discectomy, osteophytectomy, and fusion for nerve root decompression if indicated by history, examination and MRI.

NON-SPINAL BACK PAIN AND SCIATICA

Back Pain Mimics
1. Sacral chordoma, large, shown on sagittal views of MRI of normal lumbar spine; and any abdominal cancer.

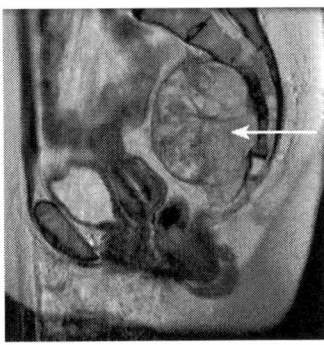

Sciatica Mimics
1. Hip joint arthritis. Usually presents with groin pain, but nearly as frequently with buttock pain mimicking sciatica or anterior thigh pain mimicking femoralgia. Good reason for routine pelvis AP view with lumbar spine x-rays.

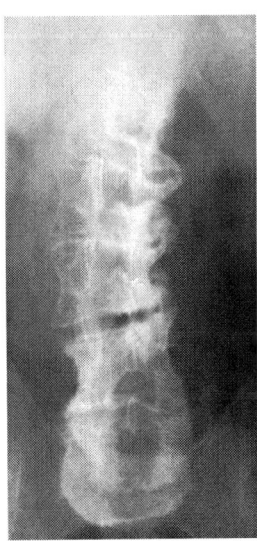
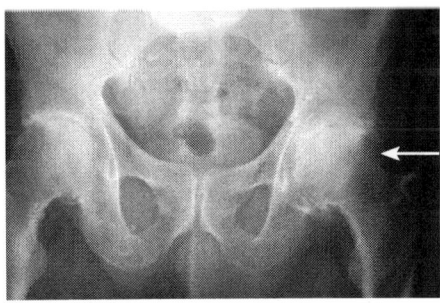

Elderly patient with severe left buttock and thigh pain. No back pain. Advanced OA left hip. MRI lumbar spine proved no neural compression, in spite of severe spondylosis on plain x-ray.

Non-Spinal Back Pain and Sciatica

2. Pelvic fracture. Elderly lady presented with "sciatica" after fall onto buttocks. Plain film of pelvis revealed fresh fractures of superior and inferior pubic rami (arrowed).

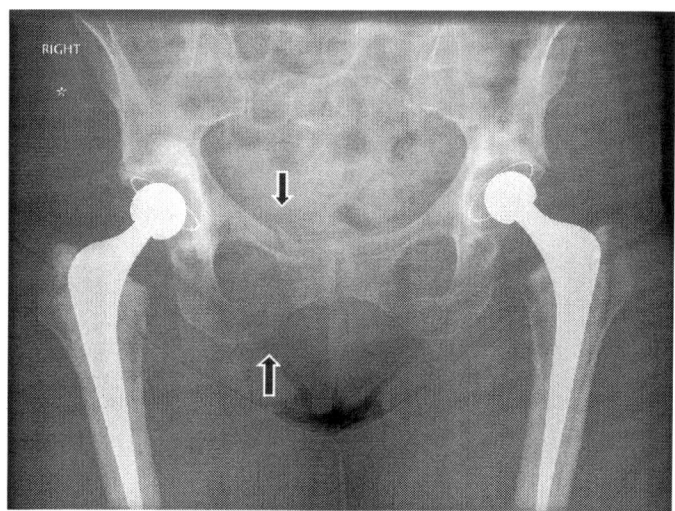

3. Hamstring strain at origin. Sports injury, especially in cricket fast bowlers. Pelvis x-ray may show avulsed bony fragment from ischial ramus but in the absence of radiological findings and a normal MRI, the give-away is marked tenderness on palpation of the ischial ramus on the affected side.

4. Trochanteric bursitis: frequent painful and very tender area at lateral prominence upper thigh, often bilateral and suffered mostly by middle aged females. Thought to be caused by inflammation in the bursa over the greater trochanter of the femur. Diagnosed on history and examination. MRI will exclude serious disease but will only rarely show fluid in the bursa. Treatment is by local infiltration with steroid and lignocaine, repeated as required if chronic.

OSTEOMYELITIS

1. Classification: several possibilities, but clinical pragmatism suggests:-
   - Acute = pyogenic = "pus forming" eg Staph, E Coli, Strep.
   - Chronic = granulomatous = "inflamed nodules" eg TB, (Brucella and Fungi = rare).

2. Anywhere in spinal column from C1 to S1 and sacroiliac joints, starting in anterior corners of vertebral bodies and quickly invading the intervertebral disc.

3. Spread by blood circulation (haematogenous) from primary infection elsewhere: lungs, teeth, ears, skin.

4. Susceptibilities: diabetes, AIDS, urinary tract procedures, renal dialysis, juveniles and aged, blood dyscrasias.

Presentation
- Acute: (eg Staph) sudden onset, severe spinal pain aggravated by movement; rigid spine; pyrexia, rigors, malaise; neurological deficit (paralysis may be sudden).
- Chronic: (eg TB) insidious onset; spinal pain aggravated by movement but less intense than in acute; night sweats; malaise; groin swellings (psoas abscesses); haemoptysis; neurological deficit (paralysis by degrees).

Differential diagnosis
- In juveniles: trauma.
- In aged: cancer, especially metastasis.

Pathophysiology (conjectured)
- Bacteraemia from primary focus anywhere (haematogenous), and frequently unknowable, but also dental, middle ear, pharynx, skin, lung (including old TB **Ghon** lesion reactivation), renal/urinary system especially after invasive investigations.

Osteomyelitis

- Bacteria colonise where blood moves slowest (venules anterior superior or inferior vertebral bodies); pus then spreads deep to anterior longitudinal ligament to adjacent disc and vertebral body.

Diagnosis
- Plain x-ray spine: (page 57,58) disc space collapse with "moth-eaten" end pates and ragged destruction of adjacent surfaces of vertebral bodies; implies some degree of disc infection as well. **Aphorism: "bad disc, good news" ie infection preferable to cancer, (where disc is normal)** (Page 58). Check for loss of psoas shadow alongside lumbar spine (psoas TB abscess).
- Plain x-ray chest: exclude pulmonary tuberculosis; exclude "heart within the heart" ie TB abscess of thoracic spine.
- MRI confirms infection rather than cancer BUT appearances in bone can be similar; shows true number of vertebrae infected; shows possible paravertebral or epidural abscess, or granulomatous compression of cord. High signal in disc space on T2 and fat suppression sequences (page 67). Vertebral marrow = dark in T1 and bright in T2 (see Table Modic page 108).
- Blood: high ESR, CRP, White cell count (differential for acute versus chronic); anti-staph and anti-strep titres; blood culture (aerobes and anaerobes) and sensitivity.
- Biopsy: histology and culture, to exclude cancer and to show acute versus chronic; may reveal organism in culture, and antibiotic sensitivity.
- Radio-isotope scan reveals spinal "hotspot" or "blackspot" (Page 59), and bone infections distant from spine, if any.

Treatment
- Chemotherapy (antibiotics) based on organism culture and sensitivity, starting intravenously for first week at least. May require **PICC** line. Monitor progress on white cell count, ESR, CRP, temperature, general condition, repeat x-rays and MRI. (CRP responds early; ESR late). Change antibiotic if response not positive within days (pyogenic) or weeks (TB). MRSA requires vancomycin or linezolid straight off,

(at time of writing). Check TB patient for AIDS and associated organism resistance.
- Chemotherapy where sensitivity not found but infection suspected to be pyogenic: combination of anti-staph and anti-coliform antibiotics eg flucloxacillin and gentamicin, plus metronidazole for anaerobes. Many variations possible. Check BNF or MIMS for dosage.
- Chemotherapy for suspected TB: Rifampicin 600mg, Isoniazid 300mg, Pyrazinamide 2 Gm; daily dosage for adults, 6-9 months. Check BNF or MIMS for refinements.
- Surgery indications:
    1. Progressive neurological deficit.
    2. Abscess.
    3. Progressive deformity.
    4. Intractable pain.
    5. Failure to respond to chemotherapy.
- Commonly required for TB.
- Rarely required for pyogenic: staph can heal with useful ankylosis.
- **Pyogenic epidural abscess shown on MRI = one of the few surgical emergencies in spinal disorders.**
- Surgical procedures: incision and drainage of paraspinal or epidural abscess; anterior vertebrectomy and fusion in TB with anterior cord compression. Iliac crest tricortical strut graft highly successful even in pyogenic infection. With infection dormant, late mechanical pain and progressive kyphosis may require surgical stabilisation. Posterior approach avoids need to open chest = costo-transversectomy (**Capener**).

Prognosis:
Paralysis in pyogenic infection is sudden and permanent. Paralysis in TB is insidious and can recover remarkably after surgical decompression of cord.

OSTEOPOROSIS

Relevance Vertebral wedge compression fractures, especially in older post-menopausal women and in the upper thoracic spine, frequently with intractable spine pain and thoracic girdle pain.

Definition Reduced bone mineral density **(BMD)** or subnormal quantity of bone per unit volume to the point where the bone is at risk of fracture in normal daily use, *but where there is a normal balance between matrix (osteoid) and mineral (calcium).* Distinguish from **osteomalacia** where subnormal quantity of bone per unit volume is associated with *reduced mineralization* of matrix. Usually dietary problem: insufficient calcium intake associated with malnutrition in third world. Some elderly women manifest both osteoporosis and osteomalacia.

WHO definition: more than 2.5 standard deviations below the mean **BMD** of healthy young adult = "T" score. Comparison with mean BMD for healthy adults of like age, gender, race = "Z" score.

Risk factors Caucasoid, post-menopausal female, positive family history, reduced physical activity, malnutrition, excessive alcohol, smoking, corticosteroid medication, primary hyperparathyroidism.

Problem Potential for intractable spinal pain and **kyphosis** deformity of vertebral fracture. Also risk of fracture neck of femur, distal radius, ribs. Pain is multifactorial: multiple trabecular microfractures; posterior ligament strain of kyphosis; girdle pain if segmental intercostal nerves compressed. However, cord compression very rare.

Diagnosis Screening programmes using **DEXA** scanning of spine, wrist or neck of femur. Clinical suspicion in elderly women with thoracic spinal pain and kyphosis. Plain x-ray of spine confirms. Biochemistry and haematology usually normal, but serum calcium raised in hyperparathyroidism.

Treatment Calcium and Vitamin D supplements; hormone replacement therapy **(HRT)**; **calcitonin; bisphosphonates**. **Vertebroplasty** for fresh vertebral fractures: injection of fast-setting acrylic pastes through pedicles to halt further deformity; and **kyphoplasty** to correct deformity by similar technique.

Prevention HRT at menopause; exercise; balanced diet. Little defence against genetic predisposition.

Osteoporosis

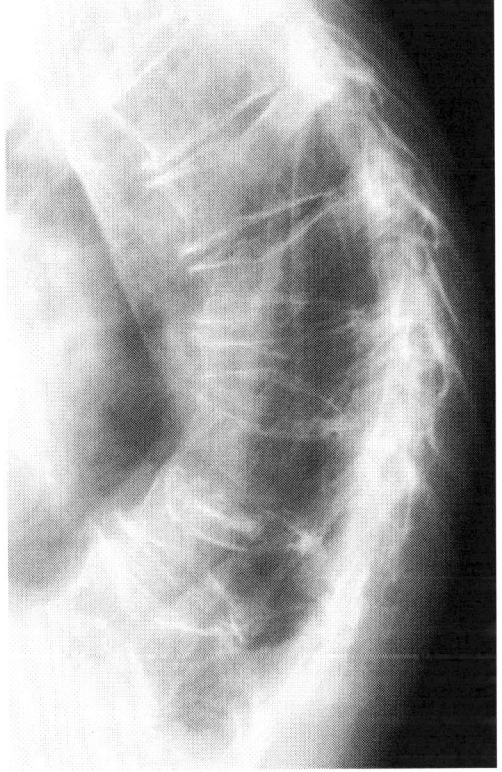

Anterior   Posterior

Thoracic spine lateral plain x-ray.
Six successive vertebrae demonstrate anterior wedging plus dishing of endplates.

OSWESTRY DISABILITY INDEX [ODI]

Was devised in 1976 by the author and Judith Couper, occupational therapist, at the Robert Jones and Agnes Hunt Orthopaedic Hospital, at the behest of the then chief of Spinal Disorders service, John O'Brien. Its design was based on clinical experience, intuition, and inspired "thumbsuck". Only much later was it validated by others, and initially by the MRC project seeking to compare hospital physiotherapy with chiropractic in the treatment of low back pain. With little modification it has survived as the most used measurement of disability in back pain, world wide. It has been altered by professional colleagues to suit application to other anatomical areas and conditions causing musculoskeletal disability.

The ODI is not an objective measure of disability. It was intended to measure the effect of an individual's pain on that individual's daily life activities, as the nearest substitute for measuring actual pain. It is not possible to measure pain itself. No measure which depends on patients' responses to questions about their pain, can be considered objective. The ODI remains a subjective "self-report" instrument with all the expected shortcomings of a measure based upon an individual's perception. There is no score which can be generalised across the population to define "mild", "moderate", or "severe" pain, nor is there a score which can be used to justify some surgical procedure.

The usefulness of the ODI is confined to the assessment of an individual patient's pain at intervals over time and during which time there may have been therapeutic interventions, including surgery.

The Index is divided into 10 categories of daily life activity, each category carrying a maximum severity score of 5. The total score is therefore a proportion of 50, but doubled so as to be scored out of 100 as a matter of cultural convenience. The score is calculated out of a smaller possible total if there is a need to exclude one of the categories.

The Index pioneered the performance of sexual activity as one of the measures of disability. Considerable dismay was expressed by professional colleagues at the first public presentation of the Index in the summer of 1976.

THE OSWESTRY DISABILITY INDEX FOR LOW BACK PAIN

The Robert Jones and Agnes Hunt Orthopaedic Hospital
Oswestry, Shropshire UK.

This "instrument" is a self-report measure of DISABILITY through back pain, relevant only to the individual who completes the questionnaire, to serve as a measure of progress (or lack thereof) for that particular patient over time and possibly through a treatment programme. The need for such a disability index arises from the impossibility of measuring pain itself. The ODI score is particular to each patient and does not pretend to place a patient at a point somewhere in the human population.

Calculating the score:-
Each SECTION is scored in the boxes 0-5, where the first option represents 0 and the sixth option represents maximum disability 5. The total is calculated out of 50, and multiplied by 2 to provide a "percentage". Where a whole SECTION is irrelevant to a patient, then the score of 5 for that SECTION is removed from the possible total.

NAME .... DATE ....

ADDRESS ....
....

DATE OF BIRTH .... AGE........................

OCCUPATION ....

I have had BACK pain for ..... years .... months ..... weeks

I have had LEG pain for   ..... years .... months ..... weeks

Oswestry Disability Index

SECTION 1 – PAIN INTENSITY
- ☐ My pain is mild to moderate: I do not need painkillers.
- ☐ The pain is bad, but I manage without taking painkillers.
- ☐ The pain is bad, but painkillers give complete relief.
- ☐ The pain is bad, and painkillers give moderate relief.
- ☐ The pain is bad, and painkillers give very little relief.
- ☐ The pain is bad, and painkillers have no effect.

SECTION 2 – PERSONAL CARE (washing, toilet, dressing)
- ☐ I can look after myself normally without causing extra pain.
- ☐ I can look after myself normally but it causes extra pain.
- ☐ It is painful to look after myself; I have to be slow and careful.
- ☐ I need some help but manage most of my personal care.
- ☐ I need help every day in most aspects of self care.
- ☐ I do not get dressed; wash with difficulty; and stay in bed.

SECTION 3 – LIFTING
- ☐ I can lift heavy weights (medium full suitcase) without extra pain.
- ☐ I can lift heavy weights but it gives me extra pain.
- ☐ I cannot lift heavy weights off the floor; I can lift off the table.
- ☐ I can lift light weights only (full kettle; briefcase).
- ☐ I can lift only very light weights (one small bag of shopping).
- ☐ I cannot lift or carry any extra weight at all.

SECTION 4 – WALKING
- ☐ I can walk as far as I wish.
- ☐ Pain prevents me walking more than 1 mile.
- ☐ Pain prevents me walking more than ½ mile.
- ☐ Pain prevents me walking more than ¼ mile.
- ☐ I can walk only if I use a stick or crutches.
- ☐ I am in a bed or in a chair for most of every day.

SECTION 5 – SITTING
- ☐ I can sit in any chair as long as I like without having extra pain.
- ☐ I can sit in my favourite chair only, as long as I like.
- ☐ Pain prevents me from sitting more than 1 hour.
- ☐ Pain prevents me from sitting more than ½ hour.
- ☐ Pain prevents me from sitting more than 10 minutes.
- ☐ Pain prevents me from sitting at all.

Oswestry Disability Index

SECTION 6 – STANDING
- ☐ I can stand as long as I want without extra pain.
- ☐ I can stand as long as I want, but with extra pain.
- ☐ Pain prevents me from standing for more than 1 hour.
- ☐ Pain prevents me from standing for more than ½ hour.
- ☐ Pain prevents me from standing for more than 10 minutes.
- ☐ Pain prevents me from standing at all

SECTION 7 – SLEEPING
- ☐ Pain does not prevent the sleep I need.
- ☐ I need some painkillers to get the sleep I need.
- ☐ Even with painkillers I get less than 6 hours sleep.
- ☐ Even with painkillers I get less than 4 hours sleep.
- ☐ Even with painkillers I get less than 2 hours sleep.
- ☐ Pain prevents me from sleeping at all.

SECTION 8 – SEX LIFE
- ☐ Normal for me; no extra pain.
- ☐ Normal for me but causes extra pain.
- ☐ Nearly normal for me but painful.
- ☐ Much restricted by back pain.
- ☐ Severely restricted by back pain.
- ☐ Pain prevents any sex life at all.

SECTION 9 – SOCIAL LIFE
- ☐ Normal for me; no extra pain.
- ☐ Normal for me but causes extra pain.
- ☐ Still regular for me but the more physical activities (eg dancing) no longer possible.
- ☐ Restricted by back pain; I do not go out as often as previously.
- ☐ Restricted to social life at home; back pain prevents me going out.
- ☐ No social life because of back pain.

SECTION 10 – TRAVELLING
- ☐ I can travel anywhere without back pain.
- ☐ I can travel anywhere but it causes extra pain.
- ☐ I cannot manage journeys lasting over 3 hours.
- ☐ I cannot manage journeys lasting over 1 hour.
- ☐ I cannot manage journeys lasting over ½ hour.
- ☐ I cannot travel at all except to the doctor or hospital.

PARALYSIS
AND
SPINAL CORD INJURY [see TRAUMA]

PHYSIOTHERAPY

- Probably most used non-surgical treatment for spinal pain, after standard analgesics.
- Has important place also in spinal post-operative rehabilitation; critical importance in rehabilitation after spinal cord injury; in scoliosis for supervision of brace wearing.
- Advantage: Multiple techniques available, free at point of delivery (in NHS); whereas chiropractic and osteopathy are restricted to fewer modalities and for a fee. (Osteopathy and chiropractic advantages: no waiting; pleasant premises; individual attention by one clinician; especially effective for neck and back strains; no parking charges).
- Techniques for spinal pain: various massages/manipulations; heat/cold; "electrics" (interferential current, shortwave diathermy, TENS provision and advice etc); exercise recommendations; hydrotherapy; acupuncture.
- No place in sciatica where lumbar disc prolapse suspected.
- No place in cervical radiculopathy or myelopathy.
- Sudden wrenching rotational manipulations should be forbidden for any spinal condition in any kind of practice.

PSEUDARTHROSIS

Literally: false joint. Persistent back pain after spinal fusion surgery can have several origins but the most likely is failure of the bone transplant (graft) to consolidate across all relevant fragments. By universal convention, a lumbar fusion should be given 12 to 18 months to prove itself, and a cervical fusion 2 to 3 months, irrespective of technique (see also p. 44).

[see also COMPLICATIONS and CONSENT]

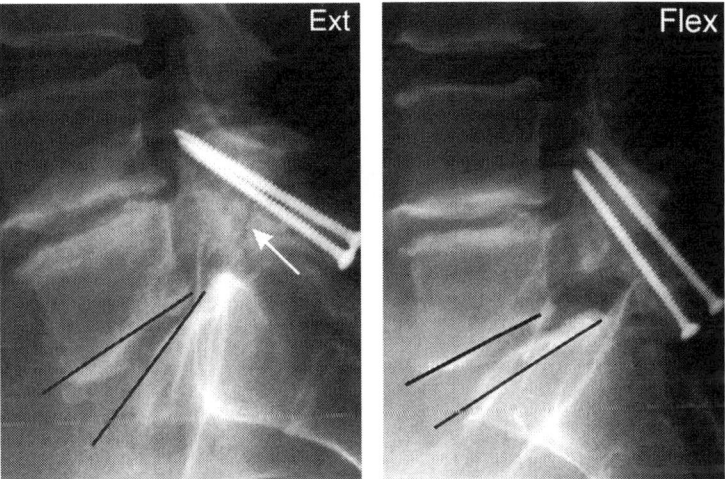

Intended posterior fusion L5/S1.
Persistent post-operation pain. Plain x-rays bending backwards (Ext) and forwards (Flex) show changing relative positions of L5/S1 end plates and fine defect in fusion mass (arrow).

POSTURE

- There is no such thing as correct posture except on the parade ground, training for ballet, preparing to be a debutante, partaking in equestrian competitions, engaging in the practice of Tai Chi, Alexander technique, and others. This statement is counter to the conventions of physiotherapy, chiropractic, and osteopathy practice. The convention of some sort of "correct" posture (upright, chest out, chin up/down, square shouldered) probably has its origins in the military, going back centuries, and based on a perception of some sort of military aesthetic.

- In spite of a widespread and unquestioning acceptance throughout western cultures of the validity of "correct" posture, there is no clinical evidence to fix blame for any disease or damage on any kind of "incorrect" posture, let alone spinal damage. Idiopathic adolescent scoliosis (curvature of the spine) is a painless condition in spite of constant "incorrectness" of posture, for the duration of the patient's life, until the changes of spondylosis supervene, as they do for all of us.

- The spine is an elastic structure. It is the whole point of spinal elasticity that the spine can adopt a variety of postures through each day and night. The question must then arise as to which of these is "incorrect" on the basis of some anticipated harm. It is highly unlikely in any event that one particular posture will be maintained for any dangerously lengthy period, unless one is dealing with a moribund bedbound invalid.

- **It must surely be the case that the only sensible posture is the most comfortable one at any one moment in the day for a particular individual. Discomfort rather than correctness or aesthetics will dictate the need to change posture. Likewise, there is no "correct" mattress beyond greatest comfort for the individual.**

- Heavy lifting is a powerful cause of low back strain and associated pain. There is certainly some posture advice to be given to those unavoidably engaged in heavy lifting: draw object close to you; never snatch; tense all muscles; lift slowly with knees slightly flexed; share the load when ever possible.

SCIATICA
[see also GLOSSARY and JARGON]

Definition Medical jargon for lower limb pain, with the unspoken expectation that the cause will be proved to be nerve root compression or irritation somewhere in the lumbar region. Lower limb pain frequently combined with numbness and tingling.
- The most common cause of nerve root compression is a disc prolapse.
- Rarely, the sciatic nerve is subject to entrapment or compression anywhere along its pathway through the pelvis. Pelvic tumours and entrapment by the piriformis muscle (the controversial "piriformis syndrome") need to be excluded by pelvic MRI if lumbosacral imaging fails to explain a sciatic presentation.
- The vast majority of disc prolapses occur at the lower two segmental levels L4/5 and L5/S1.
- Prolapses causing root compression at L3/4 and L2/3 will most likely present as **femoratica**.
- The vast majority of patients who suffer from nerve root compression in the lumbar region will present with pain in the buttock and lower limb of such intensity as to overshadow any accompanying low back pain.
- Too often, clinicians will call all lower limb pain "sciatica" when in fact it may represent "referred" or "overflow" pain (see **Referred pain** below).

Examination   Positive findings which can support the suspicion of nerve root compression are one or more of the following:-
- Stance with painful limb flexed at the knee.
- Inability to stand on tiptoe on painful side (combination of pain and S1 weakness of plantar flexors).
- Inability to do heelstand with toes elevated on painful side (L4/L5 weakness).
- Inability to lie recumbent without keeping painful limb flexed at the knee.

Sciatica

- Limited straight leg raising (SLR) on painful side PROVIDED LIMITATION IS RESULT OF PAIN AND PARAESTHESIAE IN SCIATIC DISTRIBUTION – **ask patient every time where the pain is: backache can also limit SLR significantly.**
- Weakness on resisted dorsiflexion at ankle joint ("foot drop" L4/L5), or plantar flexion (S1), or big toe extension (L5).
- Diminished sensation big toe and dorsum of foot (L4/L5); lateral border or sole of foot (S1).
- Routine search for **Clonus** and **Babinski** signs in all "sciatica" patients may yield a surprising discovery of upper motor neurone disease (spinal cord or brain).
- Routine search for pedal pulses will yield occasional arterial obstruction as an explanation for the "sciatica".

Referred pain
- Patients with low back pain of some severity will frequently complain of some pain of *lesser* severity in the lower limb (usually confined to the thigh).
- This pain usually fluctuates in tandem with the back pain as the back pain fluctuates in severity.
- Direct questioning is often necessary to extract this information. Confirmation may be achieved by asking the "opposite question": whether the patient suffers from significant lower limb pain when there is no low back pain, and achieving "NO!" in answer.
- Clinicians who suspect that they are not dealing with nerve root compression will call this "referred pain", possibly quite correctly but leaving the patient none the wiser as to what is happening to them.
- The mechanism of referred pain is still not well understood but may represent some sort of *overflow* of excessive pain input, with pain perceived in some adjacent anatomy.
- Angina with chest pain spreading or overflowing into the left arm, is an apt analogy.
- Most patients (and clinicians) will accept the *overflow* terminology with less puzzlement than the *referred pain* terminology.

- Because mechanical low back pain (and associated lower limb overflow pain) is so much more common than the sciatica of nerve root compression, overflow pain is statistically far more likely than "sciatica" as a clinical presentation.
- Clinicians who are mystified by the absence of localising neurological signs in a patient whose lower limb pain (through habit) has been labelled "sciatica", are victims of their own abuse of language. Unfortunately, they may blame their patients for demonstrating inconsistency and lack of sincerity.

Investigations
- Plain x-ray may show only some loss of disc height at one or more of the lower three lumbar segments.
- Proof of nerve root compression to fit the clinical presentation of sciatica will require myelography/CT scan at least, but ideally MRI (see p.36). The most common cause of sciatica is a prolapsed disc.

Treatment
- Gradations of intensity of treatment are available, depending on the severity of pain and associated disability.
- Oral standard painkillers (paracetamol, cocodamol, tramadol) may be sufficient for many patients, in anticipation of a steady improvement over days or weeks. Patience is frequently rewarded by spontaneous remission.
- Epidural infiltration of a steroid+local anaesthetic mixture can provide gratifying short term relief for patients in great pain and awaiting improvement or surgery.
- Surgical excision of the prolapsed portion of disc which is found to be compressing the nerve root (discectomy), is appropriate for disabling pain refractory to other treatments and the passage of time (see also p.54).

SCOLIOSIS

Definition: A curve of the spine side-to-side (in the coronal plane) which is unnatural (structural, not just postural). Rotation of individual vertebrae about the vertical axis is so common in the commonest type ("idiopathic") that rotation is almost part of the definition. Distinguish from **kyphosis** and **lordosis**.

Classification: (roughly in order of prevalence)
1. **Idiopathic.** Most common by far. Cause unknown. Many theories. Most likely a combination of genetic, hormonal, and subtle neuromuscular factors.
Two sub-types: Early onset (before age 10 years); previously "infantile" and "juvenile".
Late onset (after 10 years); previously "adolescent".

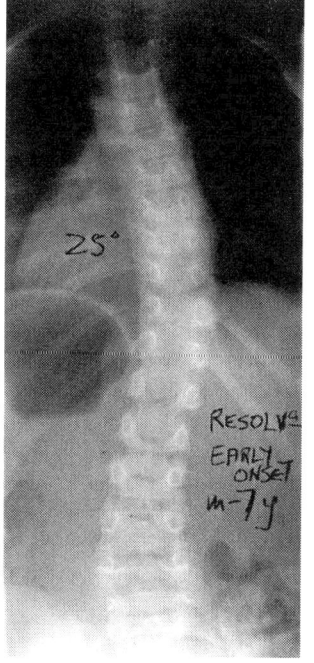

Early Onset

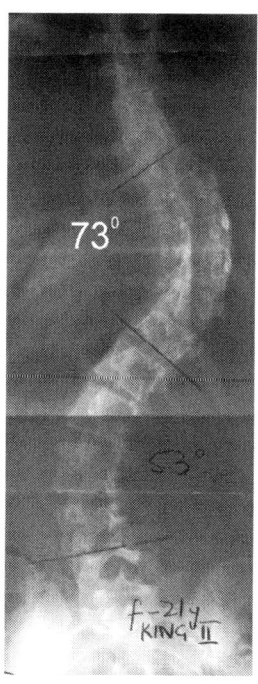

Late Onset

2. **Degenerative.** Adult and lumbar, probably a combination of undiagnosed mild adolescent idiopathic scoliosis with superimposed changes of adult **spondylosis**.

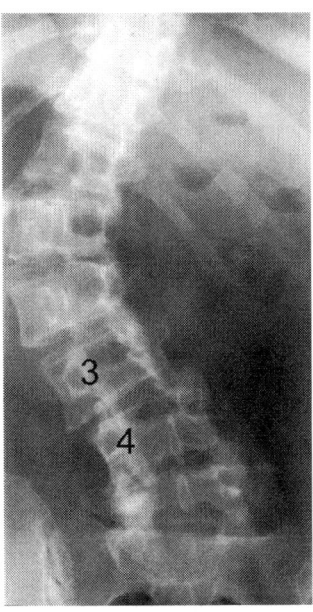

Middle-aged female presenting with intractable low back pain rather than concerns about deformity. Plain x-ray shows degenerative scoliosis. Note lateral drift of L3 off L4.

Scoliosis

3. **Congenital.** Present at birth. Not necessarily visible or diagnosable at birth.
   Two sub-types: Failure of Formation = wedge-shaped vertebrae.
   Failure of Separation = vertebrae remaining unsegmented, usually on one side.
   Can have a combination of the two types in one individual = powerful deforming force.

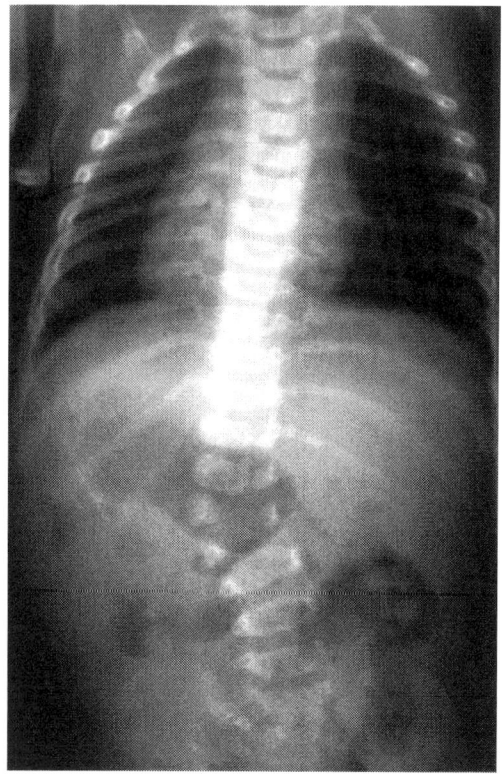

L2 is wedge-shaped and has an extra growth centre on the convexity.

4. **Neuromuscular or "Paralytic".**
   Many causes but characterised by long C-shaped curves, whether in upper or lower motor neuron cases. Cerebral palsy; myelodysplasia (spina bifida); muscular dystrophies/ atrophies (eg **Duchenne**, Fascio-scapular-humeral, Spinal Muscular Atrophy type III); poliomyelitis; tuberculosis; spinal cord injury; rare neurological illnesses eg transverse myelitis.

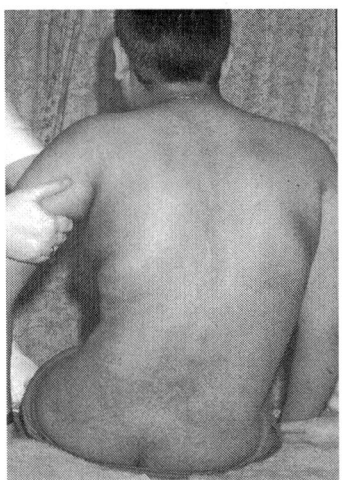
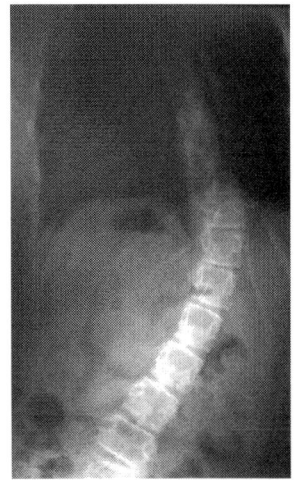

Long "C" curve typical of paralytic scoliosis (muscular dystrophy in this example). Figures show young male patient and x-rays before and after surgery.

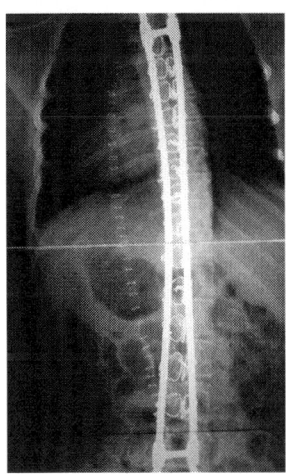

Scoliosis

5. **Traumatic.** Major violence causing asymmetric vertebral deformity.

6. **Neoplastic.** Intraspinal tumours (eg astrocytoma); vertebral or rib tumours (osteoid osteoma, osteoblastoma) may cause scoliosis with pain.

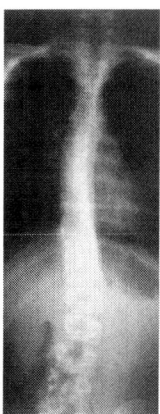 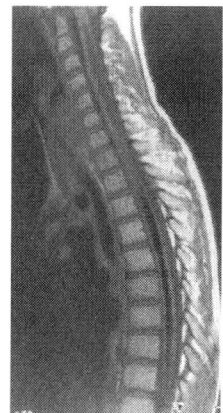 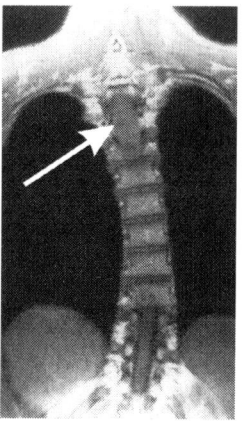

Teenager with painful scoliosis. MRI T2 lateral shows long syrinx (dark) in spinal cord.
AP X-ray shows segment of astrocytoma, upper thoracic cord. (arrowed).

7. **Inheritable Connective Tissue Disorders.**
   Rare. Autosomal dominant. eg **Marfan** syndrome; **Ehlers-Danlos** syndrome.

Scoliosis

Features and Assessment

1. **Idiopathic:**
    - Mostly adolescent girls, some with family history of scoliosis.
    - Mostly thoracic spine curves.
    - Convex right side.
    - Rib hump right side revealed on forward bending (**Adams'** Test).

    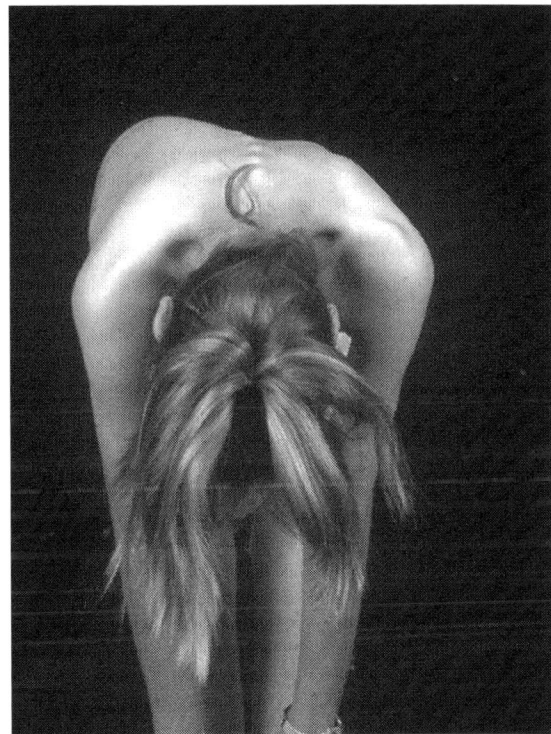

    - Shoulder girdle and waist crease asymmetry.
    - Exclude lower limb length discrepancy to save severe embarrassment and even incorrect treatment.
    - Ask about menarche.
    - PAINLESS: IF PAINFUL, LOOK FOR INTRASPINAL TUMOUR. **Red Flag!**

Scoliosis

- Plain x-ray PA (postero-anterior) standing erect whole thoracic and lumbar spine, to show iliac crests for **Risser** sign. Measure curve by **Cobb** angle. Measure rotation by **Perdriolle** goniometer. In early onset, measure rib-vertebral **Mehta** angles to judge likelihood of progressive vs resolving curves.

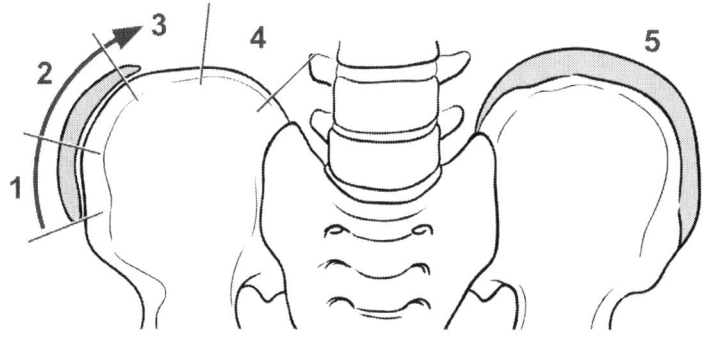

Risser Sign

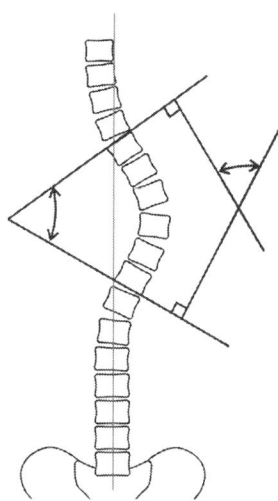

Cobb Angle

- MRI whole spine if pain a feature: idiopathic scoliosis is painless; pain may signal an intraspinal tumour.
- Plain x-ray left hand for "bone age", checked against images in atlas **(Tanner & Whitehouse)**. May be very different from chronological age.
- Contour measurements of chest wall deformity (rib hump) eg Quantec; ISIS, Oxford.
- Bending views: AP with patient supine and bending maximally to left and right, pre-operative, to reveal likely correction to be achieved with surgery.

2. **Degenerative**
   - Adult lumbar.
   - Female mainly.
   - Presents with severe back pain rather than deformity; also possibly severe subcostal nerve pain from rib cage impingement on iliac crest; also sciatica from foraminal stenosis.
   - Imaging reveals "tumbledown" spine of multilevel advanced spondylosis, scoliosis with rotation, and lateral intervertebral subluxation.

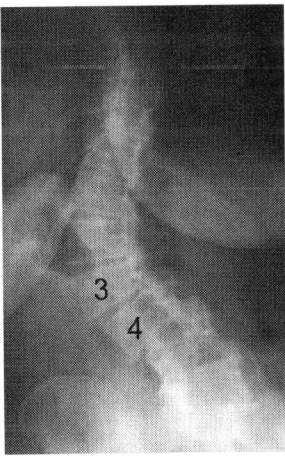

Lumbar spine plain x-ray AP.
Middle-aged woman presenting with intractable back pain. Note marked vertebral rotation as well as lateral subluxation L3 on L4 and L4 on L5 subluxation.

Scoliosis

3. **Congenital**
    - Genders equal.
    - Diagnosed usually pre-teen.
    - Postural asymmetry of spine rather than rib hump.
    - Painless.
    - Plain x-ray whole spine PA and lateral, erect: measure curves by **Cobb** method and exclude deformities elsewhere in the spine.
    - Look out for combination of wedge vertebrae coinciding with unsegmented bar.
    - MRI to exclude cord anomalies including **diastematomyelia** and **diplomyelia.**
    - Echo cardiogram to exclude cardiac abnormalities (7%).
    - IVP to exclude urinary tract anomalies (25%).

4. **Neuromuscular**
    - Most likely **Duchenne** Muscular Dystrophy (DMD), referred from a paediatric clinic.
    - Boys only, if Duchenne.
    - Check for other muscle functions esp respiration, cardiac.
    - Patients and parents will demand surgery to improve posture, handling, and setting upper limbs free for use other than trunk support.
    - Typical long curves require long fusions and fixation, if patient fit for surgery.
    - Non-Duchenne scoliosis should be fixed/fused front and back, otherwise pseudarthrosis certain, with fixation breakage.
    - Timing for surgery in Duchenne = coincidence of wheelchair and plateau of respiratory function (Yves **Rideau**).
    - Surgery characterised by copious bleeding and need for post-op assisted ventilation.
    - Duchenne boys may have cardiomyopathy: potential cause of peri-operative death.
    - All Duchenne boys will be dead at 20 years, without respiratory assistance.

5. **Trauma**
    - Spinal pain after significant traumatic event.
    - Imaging reveals deformity, probably at site of major spinal pain.
    - Indications for surgery are rare: progressive scoliosis; intractable pain at fracture site; stability for nursing and rehabilitation.
    - Neurological deficit alone is never an indication for surgery.

6. **Neoplastic**
    - Presents with painful scoliosis.
    - Tumour may be evident on MRI.
    - Mostly neural tissue eg astrocytoma but could be osteoid osteoma.
    - Rare, but a constant "red flag" worry for clinicians.

Scoliosis

Treatment

1. **Idiopathic**
    - *Non-surgical:* Regular observation and x-ray, standing, 6-12 monthly. Physiotherapy and bracing are controversial but enthusiasm for these methods remains in certain centres (Lublin, Karski; Minneapolis, Lonstein). Curves reaching 40° before anticipated maturity to be considered for surgical fixation, curve correction and fusion.
    - *Surgical:* curves 40° and over which are flexible (partially correctable by bending against the curve) can be fused and fixed posteriorly or anteriorly, depending on surgeon preference, and gratifying improvement achieved. Stiff curves require initial anterior release by transthoracic discectomy at several levels. Bewildering array of equally effective branded metal fixation systems available.
    Principle of posterior fixation = foundation "box" of pedicle screws below curve: curve pulled by hooks/wires towards rods fixed into box and rising to top of curve. "All screw" fixation gives best curve and rib hump correction.

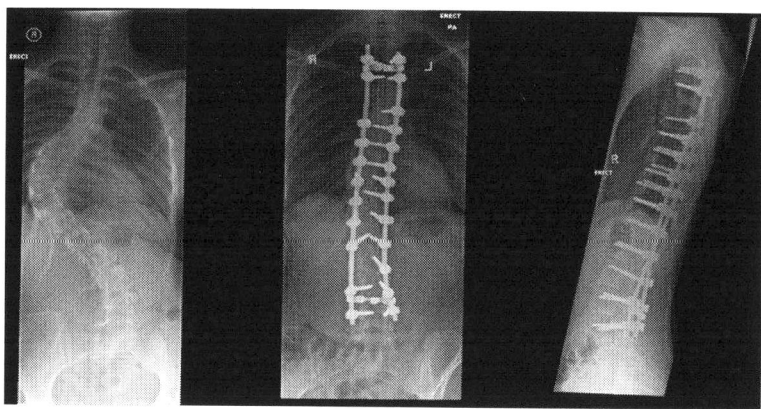

Teenager with severe scoliosis, showing excellent correction with "all-screw" fixation technique.
(Courtesy J.M. Trivedi FRCS).

Scoliosis

- **Early onset** scoliosis remains a difficult management problem: if surgery offered, must be both anterior and posterior fusion to avoid overgrowth of unfused aspect, leading to recurrence of deformity: "crankshaft".
- **Costoplasty** = most important = multilevel partial rib resection of those ribs forming hump on convex side, to diminish/obliterate rib hump.
- **King** classification of thoracic scoliosis still useful as guide to best longitudinal extent of fixation and fusion.

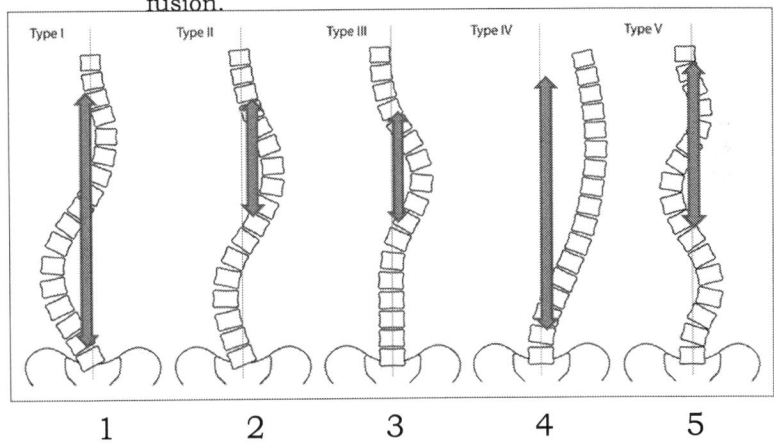

King et al. J Bone Joint Surg 1983; 65A;1302

Instrument and graft:-
King 1. Thoracic and lumbar curves.
King 2. Thoracic curve only - lumbar may correct spontaneously.
King 3. Thoracic curve only.
King 4. Thoracic and lumbar down to L4 or L5.
King 5. Usually several small curves: do thoracic curves only.

Surgery involves long procedures after exhaustive consenting process. Spinal cord monitoring throughout. Blood transfusion. Femoral head allograft. Post-operative intensive care monitoring. Seldom necessary to brace or cast for mobilisation.

Scoliosis

2. **Degenerative**
    - Rare older patient with good bone, high motivation, and in good health, justifies long fusion T10 to pelvis, restoring lumbar **lordosis** and lifting rib cage off iliac crest.

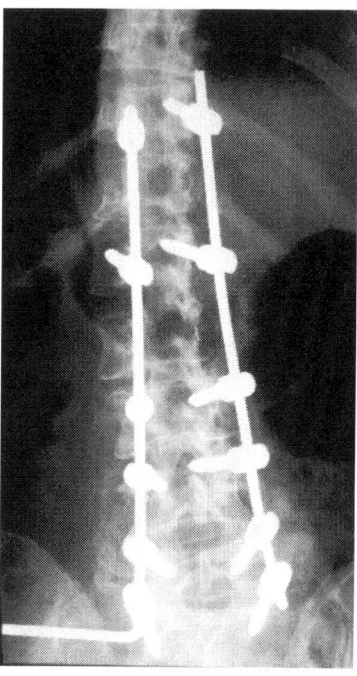

3. **Congenital**
    - *Non-surgical:* Close observation and x-ray 4-6 monthly. Bracing pointless. Assume all curves will progress. Proof of progression (typically 3 successive x-rays) justifies fusion surgery, irrespective of age. Most children will come to surgery before adolescence.
    - *Surgical:* Principle = do appropriate damage to convex side of curve, anterior and posterior, to allow correction with growth.
    Do NOT attempt correction at surgery: associated with high risk of paralysis.

Scoliosis

4. **Neuromuscular**
    - Fixation and fusion anterior and posterior imperative, except for Duchenne: posterior alone is sufficent.
    - High technical failure rate without anterior control of apex of curve.
    - Anterior surgery = discectomy and vertebral body transverse screws holding rods or plate.
    - Posterior surgery extends from high thoracic spine to pelvis.
    - Expect major blood loss.
    - Duchenne needs posterior fusion only because of low level activity and short life expectancy.
    - Post-op intensive care for cardio-respiratory function.

5. **Trauma**
    - Remember: indications for surgery have NOT to do with neurological recovery where paraplegia/ quadriplegia is complete (**Frankel A**).
    - Anterior fusion and fixation always best, whether cervical, thoracic, or lumbar.
    - Opportunity also to decompress cord: bone and disc fragments compress from anterior.
    - Where MRI shows "front-to-back" shredding of soft tissues, consider additional posterior fixation/fusion.

6. **Neoplastic**
    - Treatment is that of tumour itself, including surgical excision and/or biopsy.
    - Surgery for scoliosis required on its merits.

Scoliosis

Complications of Treatment

...are the complications of surgery:

- Most dreaded = paraplegia of varying degrees because of direct cord/ cauda equina injury or unsuspected vascular injury (anterior spinal artery; medullary feeder artery) associated with correction of deformity during operation. Spinal cord monitoring gives earliest warning of impending disaster but even this warning may be inadequate. ***Risk is 5.5/1000. Delank KS et al. Arch Orthop Trauma Surg 2005, 125: 33-41.***
- All the complications of any spinal fusion and the required surgical exposures: pseudarthrosis, instrument failure, persistent pain, donor site pain, haemopneumothorax, **chylothorax**, intercostal neuralgia, sympathectomy syndrome, diaphragmatic hernia.
- Persistent postoperative pain most likely to be result of pseudarthrosis: clue is broken and/or loose instrumentation. Revision surgery requires repeat grafting and fixation.
- Recurrence of scoliosis through additional growth.
- "Adding on": worsening of curve above or below fused segments because of incorrect choice of number of segments to be fused (see King classification table).

Prognosis
- In most cases of idiopathic scoliosis, a safe correction of 50% of deformity angle can be achieved.
- A loss of a few degrees of correction is usual in the early days and weeks of recovery.
- Majority of patients are grateful for their improved appearance in the long term.
- Girls are concerned about effect of pregnancy on scoliosis and effect of scoliosis on labour: can be reassured on both counts. If caesarean section necessary, it would have been anyway, aside from the scoliosis.
- The surgically stiffened spine has little adverse effect on physical capabilities of adolescents.
- Duchenne patients unlikely to survive beyond 20 years without major respiratory assistance.

SPINA BIFIDA

Term loosely used to describe the whole spectrum of forms of incomplete closure of the distal (lumbosacral) end of the developing spine in the foetus. The neural tube completes normal development by the end of the third week in utero, so that if defective, this congenital defect will have been present from early in the pregnancy.

The mildest form is *spina bifida occulta* where x-ray of the spine for unrelated reasons, usually in an adult with backache, reveals a previously unsuspected bifid spinous process at one or more lower lumbar and sacral levels. The only clinical significance is a statistical association with **spondylolysis** (ref.1. p.155).

At the next level of severity are lumbosacral dimples, hairy patches, and radiological spina bifida. Not likely to be associated with any disability, and no specific treatment necessary.

The more extreme forms are evident at birth, with a large lumbosacral skin and bone defect occupied by a protruding meningeal sac (meningocoele) containing CSF and even a plaque of neural tissue (myelomeningocoele). Surgical closure of the defect with reduction of the sac is a matter of urgency in order to preserve maximum neurological function and to prevent infection. In spite of best surgical treatment, most patients at this end of the spectrum have a permanent neurological deficit: paralysis of lower limbs and perineal sphincters. The more proximal defects are associated with greater neurological deficit. These remarkably cheerful children live lives of disability characterised by incontinence, recurrent urinary tract infections, lumbosacral wound breakdown, callipers and crutches, and ultimately wheelchair reliance for mobility.

Vertically extensive spina bifida may be associated with a prominent lumbar kyphos because of the absence of posterior spinal stabilizing anatomy. In the older child, frequent wound breakdown and unacceptable appearance may justify the major procedure of **kyphectomy** and posterolateral fusion.

Spina Bifida

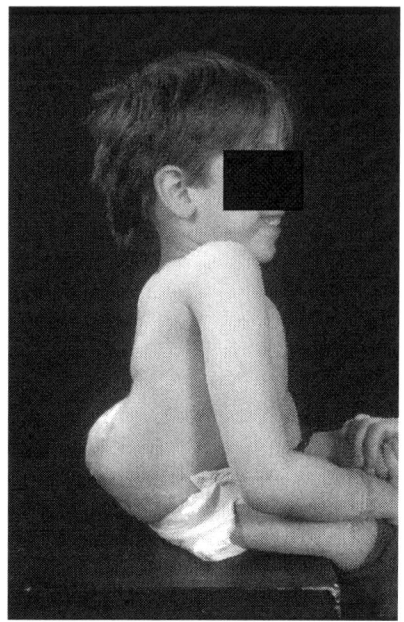

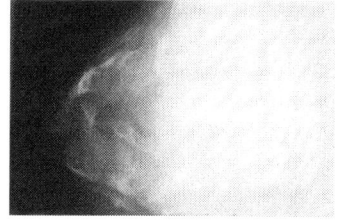

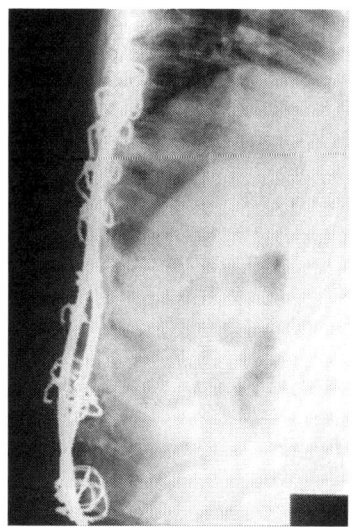

Spina bifida with paralysis and incontinence.
Note C shaped lumbar deformity and x-ray. Deformity amputated (Kyphectomy) and spine stabilised.

SPONDYLITIS

A group of unrelated or distantly related inflammatory conditions of the spine. Not to be confused with **spondylosis** which implies all the age-related changes in the spine, and where any inflammation is secondary and incidental.

Rheumatoid spondylitis
- The effect of rheumatoid arthritis on the spine.
- Can occur anywhere in the spine, causing disc degeneration, **spondylolisthesis**, endplate erosions and vertebral cyst formation not very different from infective discitis on plain X-ray.
- Presents with spinal pain and stiffness after rest, very likely in a known rheumatoid.
- Cervical spine is the area most severely affected.
- Within cervical spine, either upper cervical (occiput-C1-C2) or lower cervical (C3-C7/T1) but seldom both in the same patient, for reasons not understood.
- Upper cervical: erosion of tip of odontoid by inflammatory **pannus**, atlanto-axial subluxation, with cranial sinkage. Possible cervical myelopathy (spastic tetraparesis).
- Lower cervical: multilevel degenerative changes of disc loss with spondylolisthesis, osteoporosis, few osteophytes. Possible radiculopathy (upper limb pain, paraesthesiae, and weakness), neck pain and marked stiffness in neck.
- Thoracic and lumbar: as for lower cervical, with or without sciatica/femoralgia.
- Diagnosis seldom difficult: patient usually known rheumatoid in hands and feet. Plain x-ray of cervical spine in flexion and extension reveals movement between atlas arch and odontoid peg. Advanced premature multilevel spondylosis is another clue. MRI reveals bone destruction of tip of odontoid peg and possible impingement of odontoid remnant on anterior medulla oblongata. Serum RA latex test may be positive.
- Treatment medical: Medications and physical therapy as for rheumatoid elsewhere. Bracing in acute phases.

Spondylitis

- Treatment surgical: Spinal fusion combined, if indicated, with neural decompression. Indications for surgery are progressive or disabling neurological deficit, intractable pain, disabling deformity. Vast majority of rheumatoid spine surgery is cervical.
  Upper cervical: Transoral anterior resection of remnant of odontoid peg and **pannus** followed by posterior fusion occiput to mid or lower cervical spine with internal fixation. Warn patient that cervical spine movement in all directions will be largely lost. Preferred method of fixation = occipital plate and screws plus lateral mass screws and rods. Bone often too weak for wiring techniques.
  Lower cervical: Anterior or posterior decompression and fusion with fixation, over as many levels as considered necessary for adequate decompression and pain control.
  Thoracic, Lumbar: Decompression and fusion depending on severity of pain and neural compression.
- Complications: Prolonged steroid therapy and osteoporosis potentiate stormy post-operative course, infection, and fixation failure.

Ankylosing Spondylitis   [Syn: Marie-Strümpell d; Bechterew d.] see ANKLOSING SPONDYLITIS.

- Devastating inflammatory disease affecting spine and pelvis, including hip joints, resulting in **ankylosis** of a greater part of the spine in varying degrees of **kyphosis**. Ankylosis of hip joints less common but with forward pelvic tilt adding to kyphosis deformity.
- Develops spontaneously in young adults, usually males positive for the antigen HLA B27, with pain, stiffness, and **kyphosis** deformity in the spine increasing gradually over several years.
- One of a number of "spondylarthropathies": seronegative spine/pelvic inflammatory diseases with overlapping features. The others are: psoriatic arthritis (psoriasis, female); Reiter's syndrome (urethritis, uveitis); enteropathic spondylitis (ulcerative colitis, Crohn's disease); undifferentiated spondylitis.

- Diagnosis: In a patient apparently otherwise very well but complaining of generalised spine pain and stiffness and shortness of breath on exercise, the **Schöber** test is positive. Maximal chest excursion, measured just below nipples, is less than 5 cms. Plain x-ray may reveal actual bony ankylosis of part or whole of spine, and thoracic kyphosis. Vertebral bodies are typically squared off in lateral view, result of **enthesitis**, also known as the **Romanus** lesion. Continuity of bone over bulging intervertebral disc anulus gives "bamboo spine" appearance. <u>Earliest radiological sign is sacroiliac joint inflammatory appearance followed by ankylosis of both sacroiliac joints</u>. Serum HLA B27 positive in 95% of patients.
- Treatment non-surgical: intensive physical therapy, especially spine extension, self administered after training; anti-inflammatory medications and methotrexate.
- Treatment surgical: spinal extension osteotomy, cervical and/or lumbar, if kyphosis so severe that patient loses horizontal gaze; hip replacement for ankylosed hips fixed in flexion.
- Complications of disease: kyphosis deformity and loss of forward gaze; chest infection; spontaneous painful pseudarthrosis in one or more spinal segments.
- Complications of spinal osteotomy surgery: difficult intubation (may need tracheostomy); neural injury including tetraplegia/paraplegia during decompression and deformity correction; aortic rupture and sudden death after surgical correction of kyphosis; intra-operative haemorrhage from bone; loss of fixation because of associated osteoporosis; infection; requirement for postoperative ventilation because of poor chest excursion.
- Successful surgery produces very grateful patients. (Page 20).

SPONDYLOLISTHESIS

[G. *spondylos* vertebra + *olisthesis* slipping, falling]

Description:
   Shift, slide, or "translation" of one vertebra from its normally aligned position above the next lower or distal vertebra. Shift is usually forwards (anterolisthesis) but may be backwards (retrolisthesis) and sidewards (lateral subluxation).

Three pathological groups:
1. Degenerative (most common):
   - Based on degeneration or dehydration of the intervening disc.
   - Commonly associated with spontaneous onset chronic low back pain.
   - Middle-aged females; overweight; L4/5 ("Female, Fat, Forty, Four/Five").

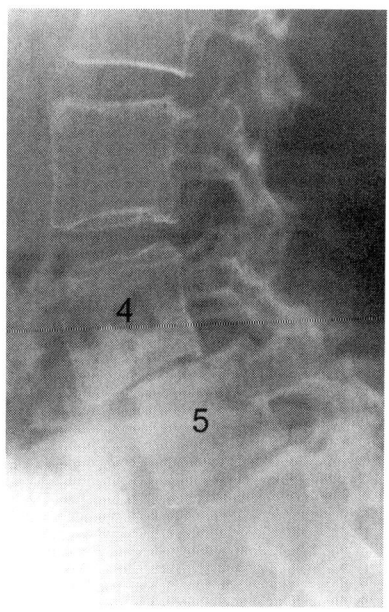

Degenerative spondylolisthesis.
L4 has slipped forwards approx 30% of the AP diameter of L5. The L4/5 disc has virtually disappeared.

- Lumbosacral segment possibly protected by tough iliolumbar ligament.
- Cauda equina rarely affected but individual nerve roots may be impinged upon by the combined effects of spondylolisthesis and spondylosis.
- Can be seen in cervical spine but rarely in thoracic spine.
- Lateral shifts are part of the picture of degenerative adult lumbar scoliosis: "tumbledown spine" (Page 136).

2. Spondylolytic ("lytic"): **See Spondylolysis.**
    - Forward shift results from fracture of pars interarticularis in childhood, revealed in adult life with onset of back pain.
    - Extent of shift is measured in Grades I – IV **(Meyerding)** or simply by estimating percentage of upper endplate of lower vertebra, uncovered.
    - Usually L5 on S1. Often associated with L5 vertebra tipping over anterior corner of sacrum ("roll over").
    - Lower limb pain is frequent association; probably combination of referred pain and L5 nerve root irritation. Presents as "tight hamstrings" on examination.

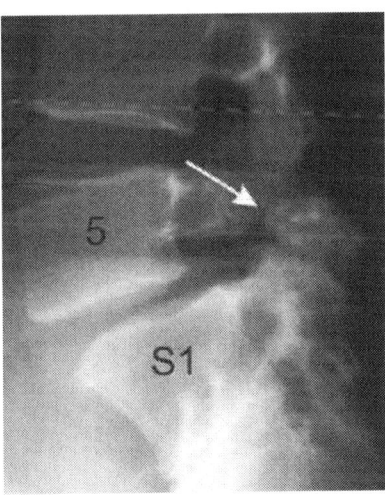

Spondylolytic spondylolisthesis.
L5 has slipped forwards on S1 approx 15% or Myerding grade 1. Arrow indicates ununited fracture ("lysis") of pars interarticularis L5.

Spondylolisthesis

- **Spondyloptosis** describes situation of vertebra shifted so far forward as to have lost support from vertebra below and tending to slide down in front of lower vertebra or sacrum.

3. Traumatic:
    - Major violence may cause such disruption of the vertebral neural arch as to allow forward shift of a vertebral body together with the rest of the proximal spine, and very likely associated with spinal cord or cauda equina damage.

Treatment:
- Of **degenerative** and **lytic**, is the management of the common presenting symptom of any back or neck pain: full trial of conservative measures.
- Strenuous reassurance: degenerative shift rarely more than 30%; after age 25, shift seldom increases.
- Rare **traumatic** spondylolisthesis will have to be managed as a spinal injury.
- If pain and disability intractable, consider for surgery: MRI preoperatively to assess proximal discs.
- Spinal fusion alone probably sufficient for degenerative.
- Fusion with excision of free neural arch L5 plus decompression L5 nerve roots required for lytic. Will need to fuse to L4 in lytic.
- Excision of the free neural arch is essential for decompression of dura and L5 roots, AND for removal of pain sources: facet joints, and lysis "ligament" with rich nerve supply.
- **Spondyloptosis** likewise, but if cosmetically unsightly, may rarely require anterior excision of L5 and some reduction of L4 onto sacrum.
- However: surgical reduction of spondylolisthesis requires massive procedures anterior and posterior, fraught with complications and mostly quite unnecessary.

SPONDYLOLYSIS
["Defect" of pars interarticularis]

1. **Is** an ununited fracture of the bony bridge between superior and inferior facet joint apophyses, usually bilateral, lower 3 lumbar vertebrae.
2. Is **not** a congenital failure of fusion of two growth centres.
3. Occurs mainly between ages of 6 and 10 years; usually asymptomatic until early adult life or later.
4. Predisposes to forward shift ("slip" or **spondylolisthesis**) of whole spine proximal to fracture.
5. Slip seldom continues after age 25.
6. Clinical problem is pain, never paralysis.
7. Prevalence is 2% to 6% depending on population[1]. Most common at L5; then L4; then L3. Rarely two or three adjacent levels in one patient.
8. **Spina bifida occulta** L5 is 6 times more common in patients with spondylolysis[1].

Clinical presentation
- Low back pain, possibly with sciatica. Back pain = non-specific; "just another back pain". Forward bending limited by reflex tension in hamstrings, "tight hamstrings".
- Back pain is likely to have many sources: all associated ligaments, anulus of disc, facet arthrosis, muscle under strain, spondylolysis ligament itself [2].
- Sciatica probably a combination of root irritation (usually L5) and referred ("overflow") pain from back.
- Visible "step" in lumbar lordosis when **spondylolisthesis** 50% and beyond.
- May be asymptomatic: incidental finding when imaging for other conditions.

Spondylolysis

Diagnosis
- Plain x-ray: lateral view may show hint of pars defect to the suspecting eye. Spondylolisthesis in adolescence or young adult is a strong indicator of possible spondylolysis.
- Plain x-ray: confirm on oblique view, showing "decapitated Scotty dog"

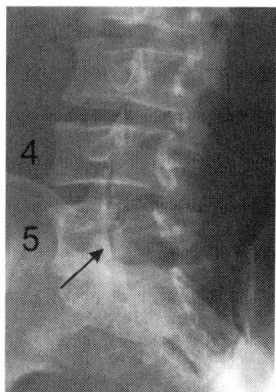 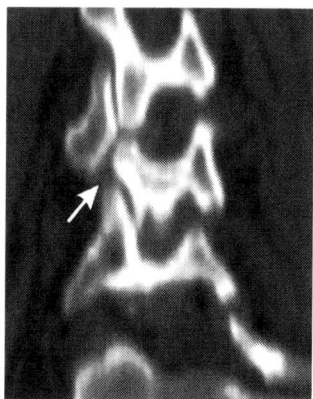

Oblique plain x-ray and CT scan show "decapitated scotty dog" L5.

- CT scan with reverse gantry: best view of defect in relation to facet joint. May also show ossified fracture debris in spinal canal affecting nerve roots in the lateral recesses.

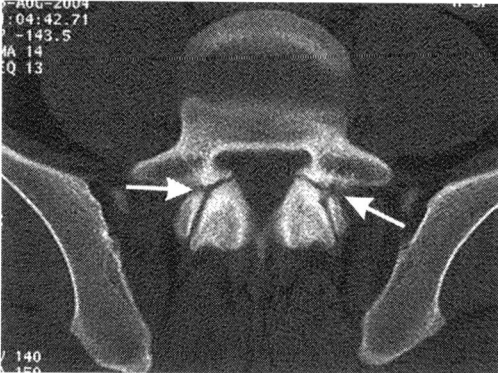

Reverse gantry or reformatted CT scan shows pars defect (arrows) as distinct from facet joints close by.

Spondylolysis

- MRI shows occasional prolapse of disc at affected level; facet hypertrophy at next proximal level; the likely dehydration of disc next proximal to the defect.

Treatment
- Non-surgical: standard analgesics and reassurance. Spinal support (corset/belt) for strenuous activity.
- Posterior Surgery for intractable symptoms in back and/or lower limbs: removal free neural arch ("rattler"); decompression of departing nerve roots; posterolateral fusion, usually with internal fixation and including level above if disc dehydrated.
- If lysis alone without vertebral shift and age less than 18 years, then consider **Scott** "butterfly" wiring and grafting of lytic defect, or **Buck** screw fusion[3], or pedicle screw/laminar hook device.

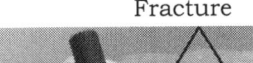
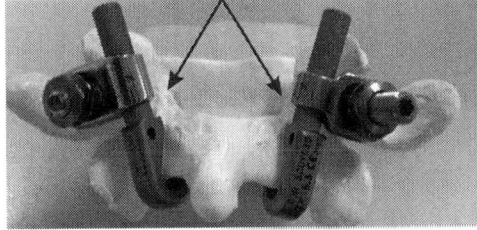

- Anterior Surgery: discectomy and fusion alone will not deal with the pain arising from spondylolysis "ligament" because neural arch is still mobile.

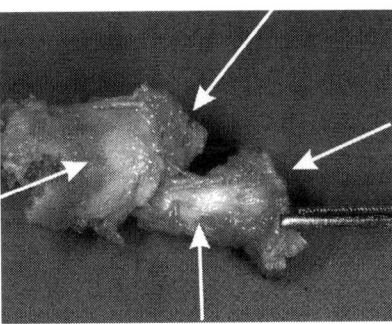

Spondylolysis

Complications
- All the complications of any spinal fusion surgery: pseudarthrosis, progressive deformity, pain, donor site syndrome, instrument failure, nerve root injury.

Prognosis
- Majority of patients grateful after surgery for less back pain and less "stiffness" in lower limbs.

References
1. *Eisenstein S. Spondylolysis. J Bone Joint Surg 60B: 488-94, 1978.*
2. *Eisenstein S et al. Innervation of the spondylolysis "ligament". Spine 19: 912–16, 1994.*
3. *Buck J. Direct repair of the defect in spondylolisthesis. J Bone Joint Surg Br 52-B:432-37, 1970.*

SPONDYLOSIS
[G. *spondylos* vertebra]

- Single word encompassing all the radiographically visible changes in a spinal motion segment associated with ageing: loss of disc height; osteophytes at vertebral body margins; sclerosis of vertebral bone adjacent to disc; enlarged and osteophytic facet joints ("lettuce leaves").
- Author prefers to refer to "wear-and-tear" in the presence of patients.
- Also called "arthritis" or "osteoarthritis" or "O/A spine" inappropriately, and causing serious fright in many patients with backache, leading them to believe they have a serious disease with a future confined to a wheelchair. Most patients can be confronted with a diagnosis of "hip arthritis" without feeling any great concern: everybody knows somebody who has had a successful hip replacement for arthritis. For cultural reasons the same cannot be said of the "A" word in respect of the spine.
- Also called "degenerative disc disease" inappropriately, unless ageing is accepted as a disease.
- May be associated with **back pain** and spinal **stenosis**; but may be incidental finding without symptoms.
- Spondylosis in certain middle-aged patients, radiologically advanced beyond expectations and painful, may be associated with a constitutional (genetic ?) predisposition to osteoarthritis: eg **Heberden's** arthropathy; characteristic swelling of distal interphalangeal joints of fingers.

	T1 MRI BONE SHADE	T2 MRI BONE SHADE	MARROW HISTOLOGY
EARLY DISC DEGEN. MODIC 1	DARK	BRIGHT	OEDEMA
LATER DISC DEGEN. MODIC 2	BRIGHT	BRIGHT	FAT
CHRONIC DISC DEGEN. MODIC 3	DARK	DARK	BONE SCLEROSIS FIBROSIS

Reference: Modic MT, Steinberg PM, Ross JS, Masaryk TJ, Carter JR. Degenerative disk disease: assessment of changes in vertebral body marrow with MR imaging. *Radiology*: 194:193-9, 1988.

STENOSIS
[narrowing of spinal canal; refers equally to clinical syndrome]

1. Usually midlumbar.
2. Genders equal; presents early 60's onwards.
3. Produced by age-related changes (**spondylosis**) in bone and soft tissues forming the spinal canal. Osteophytes and thickened ligaments cause a "Coke bottle" squeeze of the **cauda equina.**
4. Usually circumferential: **MRI** shows intrusion of facet joint osteophytes; thickened ligamentum flavum; diffuse disc bulge; intrusion of vertebral body osteophytes.
5. Developmental (genetic) narrow spinal canal will predispose to early multilevel stenosis and symptoms. Almost inevitable in **achondroplastic** dwarfism.
6. Symptoms may be unilateral i.e. stenosis involves root canal only.

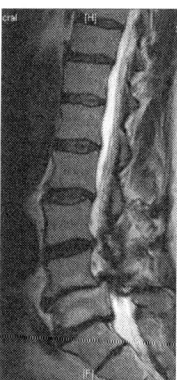

Sagittal T2 MRI:
Advanced spondylosis L4/5 L5/S1 with L4/5 spondylolisthesis and lumbar canal stenosis

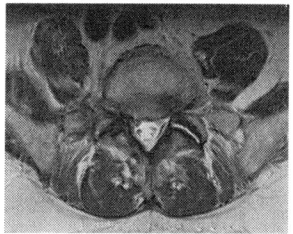 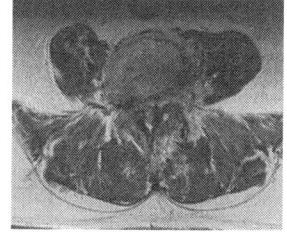

Axial T2 MRI: normal canal capacity behind L4 body (left); marked constriction of canal at L4/5 (right), multifactorial.

Stenosis

Diagnosis .... on history almost exclusively:
- Spinal **claudication** – chart: walking distance; easier up slopes than down; need to flex/sit, on reaching limit; time to recovery usually few minutes only.
- Good peripheral circulation.
- No neurological signs in lower limbs.
- Distinguish from arterial claudication: poor peripheral pulses; no need to flex/sit at claudication limit; easier down slopes than up.
- NB SPINAL CLAUDICATION AND ARTERIAL CLAUDICATION MAY CO-EXIST IN THIS AGE GROUP.
- In advanced cases: claudication distance = few yards only; urinary frequency or incontinence.
- Spastic gait and manual clumsiness suggest rare cervical or thoracic stenosis; examination reveals upper motor neurone picture. **Hoffmann** sign positive in cervical stenosis. Collectively called cervical **myelopathy.**

Investigations
- Plain x-rays of lumbar spine and pelvis: confirm spondylosis; exclude crude evidence of cancer, infection, osteoporosis.
- Ditto plain x-rays of cervical and thoracic spine.
- Arterial flow studies if circulation suspect.
- MRI : best reserved for planning surgery, if and when, and which levels.
- MRI essential for confirming diagnosis in cervical and thoracic stenosis. Altered cord signal in cervical myelopathy represents spinal cord damage and requires early cervical decompression. Ossification of posterior longitudinal ligament (**OPLL**) common in cervical spine of Japanese. Ossified disc prolapse and ossification of ligamentum flavum seen in thoracic spine.
- General health: questions and relevant tests; these patients may have concurrent diseases.

Stenosis

Treatment
- Conservative: modify lifestyle to suit circumstances; use walking trolley where possible; acquire "Disabled" badge for car.
- Surgical: decompression surgery when walking distance so short and symptoms intolerable; patient to be aware of risks of surgery in general and for patient in particular. Patient to be informed that recovery of lower limb function can continue slowly for 18 months.
- Cervical and thoracic stenosis: decompression surgery indicated on diagnosis. Patient to be warned that expectation is no more than stopping neurological deterioration.
- Operation: lumbar decompression = **laminotomy**, medial facetectomy, flavectomy, foraminotomy, discectomy, osteophytectomy. Performed at all levels required and usually both sides.
- Operation: posterior intervertebral distraction = insertion of a prosthesis between spinous processes. Simple and safe day-case procedure, gaining in popularity. Probably suitable for frail elderly and for single level stenosis only.
- Operation: cervical or thoracic decompression = anterior or posterior or both, almost always with fusion & fixation. A variety of multilevel laminoplasty techniques for relieving cervical stenosis in **OPLL.**
- Operation: lumbar fusion = additional to decompression if back pain alone is disabling; if spondylolisthesis at risk of progression; if young age raises possibility of recurrence of stenosis.

Complications
- Most feared: neurological injury = nerve root at lumbar level; spinal cord at cervical and thoracic levels. Thoracic discectomy = 20% chance of paralysis.
- All the other complications of spinal surgery: death, infection, thrombosis, painful scar, donor site syndrome.

Prognosis
- The fit elderly with lumbar stenosis and spinal claudication are some of the most grateful postoperative patients one can have after decompression surgery. "Postcard syndrome" = card from exotic holiday location indicating some remarkable distance walked, 18 months post op.
- After cervical decompression (and fusion) for cervical myelopathy in cervical stenosis, the best the patient can hope for is the status quo at time of surgery ie a halt to the progressive loss of neurological function.

SURGERY – INTRODUCTION

- There are only two operations performed for spinal disorders: **Decompression** and **Stabilisation**. On occasion, they are performed on the same patient at the same sitting. Many variations of either operation may be performed anteriorly or posteriorly.

- **Decompression is performed** to relieve neural compression, actual or anticipated.

- **Stabilisation is performed** to solidify or strengthen the spine in a wide variety of pathologies including spondylosis (pain), scoliosis (deformity), and diseases potentially destructive of the spine.

- **Until recently, "fusion" would have been the appropriate term to use** instead of "stabilisation". Fusion operations imply the use of bone or bone substitutes for transplant or grafting onto the spine. Fusion was the only means of achieving long term stability in the spine. Even in this context, the term is not quite correct: surgeons can transplant; only biology can "fuse". Customary use of the terminology allowed surgeons the flattery of calling their bone grafting operations, "fusions". A more appropriate term, as for similar operations on other joints, would be **arthrodesis.** Now there are several new techniques of binding up spinal segments to reduce intersegmental motion, or to insert artificial discs, without the need to resort to bone grafting. These techniques are used mainly for the pain of **spondylosis**. The advantage of their use lies in the avoidance of the considerable side effects associated with the harvesting of bone for grafting, and the continuing pain associated with graft failure (PSEUDARTHROSIS). It remains to be seen whether these techniques will be found to be more useful than arthrodesis, in the long term. In the meantime, "stabilisation" is an appropriate inclusive term for all those operations which are intended to strengthen segments of the spine.

- **There are no minor operations for spinal disorders**. There is never an opportunity for the spinal surgeon to "relax" concentration or reduce anxiety during an operating session by listing a couple of "minor" spinal operations for a session of surgery. Every procedure is potentially fraught with the kind of failure which could end up in the courts, with permanent damage to a professional career. Patients need to be made aware of this, hence the emphasis on an extensive consenting process (see CONSENT and COMPLICATIONS).

- **Surgery should never be an imperative, merely an offer.** For most patients potentially facing spinal surgery, their only previous experience of surgery will have been tonsillectomy, appendicectomy, or even hip replacement, all with excellent results and what the patient would consider a cure. In spinal disorders surgery, patients need to understand that:-
    1. **There is no "cure".** They should hope for merely an "improvement", especially as regards pain. A successful operation for spinal pain is one which converts unmanageable pain into manageable pain.
    2. **There is no "guarantee"** of any level of result. Most spinal operations produce "success" for 70% to 80% of patients.
    3. **No one has to have an operation.** Even a patient facing paralysis from cancer is welcome to refuse surgery. Patients who agree to have the surgery on offer, and after a full consenting process, should accept the results of the surgery (blatant negligence excepted) on the basis that they were full partners in the decision.

- **Surgery should be regarded always as an act of desperation**; a solution for the "end of the road" situation. All conservative therapies, including infiltrations, will eventually work themselves out of the system, but surgery can never be "undone". Surgeons as individuals vary considerably in their inclination to offer surgery, especially in respect of chronic pain with spondylosis. Unlike major joint replacement surgery for arthritis, there is no universally accepted scoring system for spinal disorders, where surgery is justifiably offered simply on the basis of reaching a certain score.

Surgery

- **Contra-indications to surgery for back pain** should be obvious, but are not, and are worthy of listing here:-

    1. Pending compensation claims for personal injury. As long as a successful claim for a lot of money depends on the demonstration of major disability, there is no hope of alleviating symptoms and associated disability through surgery.
    2. An insistence by the patient on a complete cure.
    3. Morbid obesity makes for difficult surgery, more postoperative complications, and a higher rate of failure to alleviate pain symptoms.
    4. More than two adjacent segmental levels requiring fusion.
    5. The profession by the patient of widespread disabling pain and tenderness combined with disability dramatically beyond any explanation by discoverable pathology.

- **Anaesthesia for Spinal Surgery.** Because most spinal operations require the patient to be in the prone position, there will be some additional anxiety for the anaesthetist and surgeon:
    1. The prone position can produce bizarre responses by the cardiovascular system.
    2. Connections to the endotracheal tube cannot be seen routinely to be intact.
    3. Poor protection of tissues can result in damage to skin, especially of face; and ulnar nerve palsies at the elbows.

    Postoperative pain can be intense, especially after spinal fusion surgery. A considerate anaesthetist will provide PCA (Patient Controlled Analgesia), and the use of the apparatus will have been explained to the patient before surgery by the anaesthetic assistants.

    Diclofenac suppositories are particularly effective in controlling postoperative bone pain, over and above the standard morphine provision.

- **Antibiotic prophylaxis** in the form of a broad spectrum cephalosporin, given intravenously at induction is appropriate in the light of the seriousness of deep infection as a complication of spinal surgery. Prophylactic antibiotics are given routinely for invasive imaging techniques of spine; more than sufficient justification for their use in open spinal surgery.

SURGERY – DECOMPRESSION

Introduction
- Whereas stabilisation operations are mostly concerned with a symptom (pain) not always supported by clearly revealed pathology, decompression operations are almost always supported by clearly demonstrated neural compression.
- The standard investigation is MRI, usually not available to the NHS practitioner in primary care because of expense and scarcity.
- Plain x-rays should always be available in preparation for surgery, especially the postero-anterior view, to reveal or exclude transitional anatomy at the lumbosacral junction. "Wrong level" surgery can be avoided.

Indications (approximate order of frequency):
1. Disc prolapse (protrusion, extrusion, or sequestration) with sciatica.
2. Spinal stenosis with claudication.
3. Root compression in cervical spondylosis.
4. Cord or cauda equina compression in metastatic disease, infection, trauma, large central lumbar disc prolapse.
5. Root compression, usually L5, in lytic spondylolisthesis.
6. Root compression by synovial cyst of facet joint.
7. Cord compression in cervical spondylosis or by ossification of ligamentum flavum of thoracic spine.

Surgery

Techniques
1. Posterior approach = for most lumbar neural compressions.
    - Laminotomy, flavectomy, medial facetectomy, discectomy: for disc prolapse single level, one side. Same for rare synovial cyst but discectomy usually not required.
    - Multilevel laminotomy, flavectomy, medial facetectomy, foraminotomy, undercutting laminar shaving, discectomy where necessary: for spinal claudication.
    - Hemilaminectomy may be necessary in spinal stenosis with advanced spondylosis, to achieve best neural release and for the sake of expedition.
    - Laminectomy = excision of free neural arch: in lytic spondylolisthesis. Laminectomy is mechanically destructive, therefore potentially weakening of that segment. Laminectomy merely for access to the spinal canal should not be necessary except for excision of neural tumours and vascular malformations.

2. Anterior approach = technique of choice:
    - For cervical discectomy and osteophytectomy, for up to three adjacent segments. For cervical spondylosis usually. For cervical myelopathy rarely.
    - For thoracic discectomy in rare thoracic disc prolapse; for thoracic spine tumours and infections; for multilevel discectomy as release in severe scoliosis. Thoracotomy with rib resection requires closure over intercostal drain bubbling through underwater seal. Anterior approach for T10/11 down to L2: probably needs to be transthoracic, trans diaphragmatic, retroperitoneal, not just for decompression but for fusion likely to follow.
    - For lumbar tumours and infections, where posterior approach not technically appropriate.

Surgery

Recovery
- Will depend on what major procedure (fusion; disc replacement) is done following the decompression, and on individual patient circumstances.
- Lumbar discectomy patients mobilise same day; discharge next day.
- Anterior decompression almost always done in preparation for something else (fusion; disc replacement): recovery determined by the greater procedure, usually not the decompression.
- Whatever approach, most patients ambulant 7-10 days postop, and encouraged to walk maximum possible, daily. Intercostal drain removed at 48 hours if lung inflated (on x-ray).
- Simple lumbar disc excision: drive 10-14 days postop; desk-bound work 6 weeks; some moderate physical strain at 3 months.
- Multilevel or combined procedures, or transthoracic: ambulation as possible; drive 3 months; deskbound work 3-6 months; no physical strain for first 12 months. Lumbar support for lumbar fusion patients, when "out and about". Debilitating diseases will delay this timetable.

Complications
Posterior approaches:
- Epidural bleeding
- Neural injury including spinal cord

Anterior approaches:
- Pneumothorax
- Haemothorax
- Chylothorax
- Empyema
- Intercostal neuralgia
- **Ileus**
- Major vessel injury
- Spinal cord injury including anterior spinal artery thrombosis

SURGERY – STABILISATION

Introduction
- The purpose of stabilisation surgery is to abolish or reduce intersegmental movement, as a pre-condition for reducing or abolishing pain, or for maintaining structural integrity after excision of diseased vertebral bone.
- Surgery in the form of spinal fusion (arthrodesis) is a final therapy of desperation, but remains the most successful treatment for refractory and intractable back pain, in the presence of identifiable pathology.
- Surgery in the form of flexible fixation without fusion ("soft fusion") is a newer stabilisation technique gaining in popularity but still controversial. No bone grafting required.
- Disc replacement is a form of stabilisation: the residual movement is less than normal, and the best results are in those patients where an inadvertent fusion takes place across the disc prosthesis (FDA multicentre trial report, Porto, Portugal, 2004).
- Segmental levels to be grafted are determined by MRI. Grafting more than two adjacent segmental levels in an adult carries a high failure rate through pseudarthrosis.
- Fixation and fusion of many segmental levels for scoliosis in adolescents is a special case: see SCOLIOSIS.

Indications
1. Intractable pain of spondylosis.
2. Progressive scoliosis.
3. Serious injury.
4. After excision of vertebral metastases or infection.
5. After decompression in lytic spondylolisthesis.
6. After osteotomy to correct kyphosis in ankylosing spondylitis.
7. For excessive intervertebral laxity with pain, in rheumatoid arthritis.

Surgery

Techniques
- All arthrodesis operations are based on the transplant of bone onto or into a bed of decorticated bleeding cancellous bone so as to bridge an existing gap between existing bone segments.
- Surgical approaches for stabilisation may be anterior or posterior, or combined, depending on surgeon's preference and experience. The best material for grafting, in terms of successful incorporation into a posterior graft bed, is autogenous cancellous bone. For anterior, autogenous cortico-cancellous bone block.
- Most common source for harvesting graft is iliac crest. Graft donor site pain is a common complication detracting from a potentially good result of surgery.
- The grafting procedure may be assisted by applying a supporting scaffolding (internal fixation), usually titanium screws, hooks, and connecting rods or plates.
- An alternative support is a strut in the form of a cage occupying the disc space, made of metal or plastic (PEEK), with space to be filled with bone graft. Cages anteriorly are ideally combined with some form of fixation posteriorly.
- Lumbar spine cages or bone blocks may be inserted by anterior approach (ALIF) or by posterior (PLIF). Latter technique developed by Ralph B Cloward, 1943 (see EPONYMS).
- For fixation without fusion ("soft fusion") and disc replacement, it is neither necessary nor desirable to decorticate down to bleeding cancellous bone.
- Fusion, when indicated, is likely to remain the standard procedure for severe back pain for some time to come. Anticipated in the near future is a bone graft substitute nearly equivalent in success to autogenous harvested bone.
- Bone graft substitutes currently in use usually consist of varying combinations of tri-calcium phosphate and calcium sulphate. Bone morphogenic protein (BMP) may be an additive, very expensive, but promising.

Surgery

Recovery
- Post-operative rehabilitation is a slow progression of physical capability but excludes all heavy lifting and strenuous physical stress for at least 12 months. Walking is beneficial from start: excellent and underrated. No driving for first two months. Spinal brace/corset for heavy or hyperactive patients, for 3-4 months.
- Surgical success judged no sooner than 12–18 months post-operatively: major gratifying reduction in pain and plain x-rays suggesting bone graft consolidation.
- Newer procedures avoiding need for bone grafting are intended to allow residual segmental motion and earlier return to physical activity. They depend on long lasting integrity of implants: eg pedicle screws attached to cables; various metal and high density polyethylene disc replacements.

Complications (see also COMPLICATIONS for risk levels and references).
All complications listed here are rare, but varyingly dramatic and serious.
Complications common to all spinal surgery are: death, paralysis, CSF leak, infection, thrombosis with pulmonary embolus, persistent symptoms, donor site pain.

Cervical:
- Recurrent laryngeal nerve palsy resulting in hoarse voice, following right side anterior cervical approach.
- Lymphocoele following damage to (invisible) thoracic duct in left side anterior cervical approach.
- Perforation of oesophagus with any anterior cervical approach.
- Injury to any of the great vessels in the neck. Most worrying is injury to vertebral artery because of difficulty of access for control of bleeding.
- Loss of anterior fixation, with oesophageal or tracheal compression, and need for surgical removal.
- Spinal cord injury with quadriplegia following anterior decompression and fusion.

Thoracic:
- Complications special to anterior approaches: injury to mediastinal anatomy; haemopneumothorax; intercostal neuralgia; spinal cord injury from misplaced anterior fixation, diaphragmatic hernia.

Lumbar:
- Retrograde ejaculation in males following undetectable injury to inferior hypogastric plexus during anterior dissection.
- Great vessel injury, especially iliac vein, with potentially major haemorrhage, during anterior approach. Injury to abdominal viscera during anterior surgery for fusion with/without fixation, and disc replacement.
- Displacement of anterior internal fixation or disc implants, requiring hazardous repeat anterior approach to rectify.
- Donor site pain syndrome in iliac crest following bone harvest for fusion graft.

All levels:
- Adjacent level degeneration. Theoretical possibility that successful fusion imposes extra strains on adjacent unfused levels, thereby accelerating degenerative changes, with symptoms. Impossible to know if relevant, as against natural history.
- Pseudarthrosis.
- Implant complications: loosening, misplacement, displacement, neural injury, vascular perforation.

Surgery

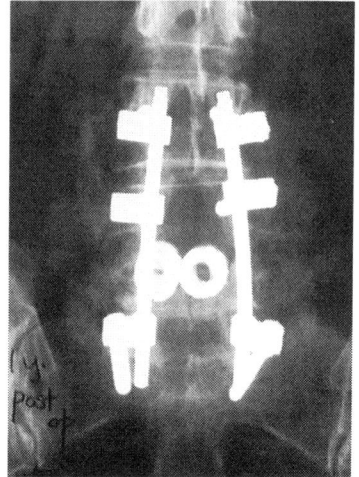 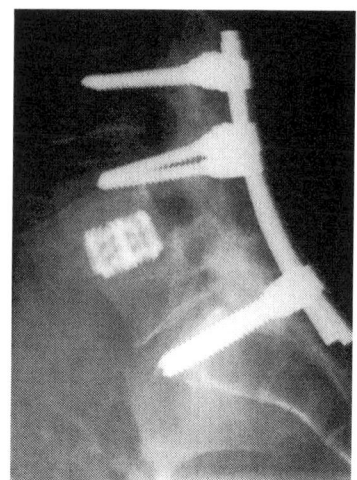

Posteriolateral fusion 1 year after operation for lytic spondylolisthesis L4/5, with pedicle screw fixation, cages in L4/5 disc space. Bone graft in paravertebral gutters.

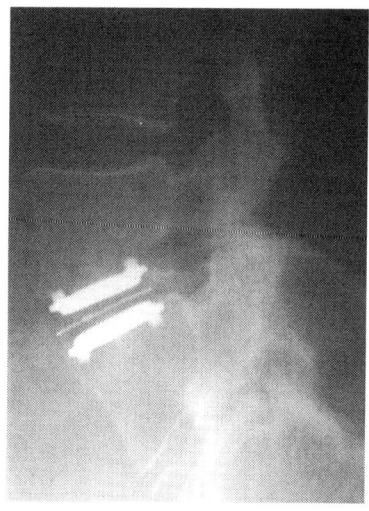

Anterior disc replacement L4/5 for painful spondylosis.

TRAUMA

1. Spinal injury can damage both the mechanical structure of the spinal column and the neural anatomy contained therein.
2. On admission, the first demand is to exclude life-threatening other injuries.
3. The next demand is to know whether or not there is a neurological deficit, and whether that is upper or lower motor neurone (cord or **cauda equina**).
4. Finally, there must be an assessment of the residual danger to the neurology by the nature of the structural injury to the spinal column ("stable" vs "unstable").
5. There is seldom any indication for emergency surgery in spinal trauma: what is considered "unstable" (danger to neurology) on arrival may be quite "stable" (safe) weeks or months later.
6. Meticulous neurological examination, early and repeated, is the beginning of good care of spinal injured patients.
7. The historical obsession with the state of the spinal column must give way to concerns for the complications of spinal cord injury: **dysautonomia**, urinary tract problems, bedsores, cardiac function [1].
8. The dogmatic highly technical definitions of indications for decompression and stabilisation surgery, so much in vogue, are probably irrelevant in reality [3,4].
9. The plain x-rays will show only the last frame of a movie. You will never get to see the movie. The damage to the spinal cord is done and no emergency surgery will undo it.
10. No proof exists that emergency decompression surgery of itself was ever responsible for a significant and useful neurological recovery, except perhaps for obvious progressive neurological deterioration.

Presentation
- <u>Conscious:</u> questioning and a brief neurological examination will quickly reveal the possibility of a spinal injury.
- <u>Unconscious with multiple trauma:</u> remember, in the intensity of life-saving activity, that there may be a spinal injury and that the vigour of resuscitation may be creating or adding to neurological deficit.

Trauma

Examination
- Spine plus: Palpation may reveal a soft gap between spinous processes, tender in the conscious patient. Unexplained forehead abrasion may signal cervical spine injury. A palpable sternomanubrial dislocation indicates a high thoracic fracture-dislocation. Percuss lower abdomen to exclude distended bladder.
- Sensation: Routine light touch throughout trunk and all four limbs, BUT pinprick distal to suspected level of injury = most important as good prognostic sign. Better still if pinprick felt peri-anal = "sacral sparing". Peri-anal and perineal anaesthesia = poor prognostic sign. Remember position sense and vibration for posterior columns. Temperature perception, for completeness and to diagnose **Brown-Sequard** syndrome.
- Power: Even a mere flicker of voluntary movement distal to injury is good prognostic sign. Document power according to **MRC** (Medical Research Council) grades. Must do rectal examination (for sensation) and anal sphincter tone: poor tone = poor prognosis.
- Reflexes: confusing in first 12 hours to 7 days of spinal cord injury; may be flaccid because of "spinal shock", converting to spastic thereafter: **clonus** and positive **Babinski**, and positive **Hoffmann** if cervical cord involved.

Summarise findings for **Frankel** classification [2]. Good chance (over 60%) that Frankel B will walk again albeit with aids, AND EVEN WITHOUT HAVING HAD SURGERY.

Alternative similar classification is ASIA IScoS (American Spinal Injury Association in association with International Spinal Cord Society) which is based on the Frankel classification but with more detail. *http://www.asia-spinalinjury.org/publications/store.php.*

FRANKEL CLASSIFICATION of NEUROLOGICAL DEFICIT in SPINAL CORD INJURY [2]

GRADE	NAME	DESCRIPTION
A	Complete	No motor or sensory function below level of injury
B	Sensory only	Some sensation present below level of injury. Complete motor paralysis
C	Motor useless	Some sensation and motor power below level of injury but no practical use to patient
D	Motor useful	Useful sensation and power below level of injury, moving lower limbs, or walking, even with aids
E	Recovery	No weakness, sensory loss, sphincter disturbance. Brisk reflexes and Babinski may be present

Investigations
- Any imaging will require patient transfers: safe transfers require many hands, slide boards, sandbags, bracing.
- Plain x-rays will reveal one or other deformity or a combination: vertebral body wedge compression; dislocation, unilateral and bilateral; fracture-dislocation; burst fracture; cervical "tear-drop" fracture. The evidence from plain x-rays is sufficient in most cases to suggest the intensity of care required in the next stage of management ie whether or not the spinal cord/cauda equina is at risk of further injury from careless handling of patient.

A LATERAL PLAIN X-RAY OF CERVICAL SPINE MUST SHOW DOWN TO T1 TO "CLEAR" THE SPINE.

- Rare: a sternomanubrial dislocation almost certainly accompanies a thoracic spine fracture-dislocation.
- Not so rare: lumbar spine transverse process fractures indicate major violence. A ruptured viscus and a retroperitoneal haematoma must be excluded.
- Evidence of injury at one spinal level: imperative to "clear" the rest of the spine.

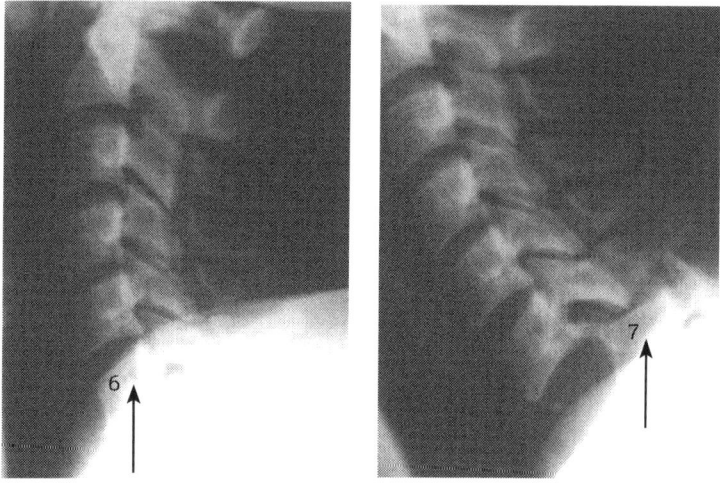

Lateral plain x-ray on left down to C6 in injured patient, fails to reveal gross fracture/dislocation C6/7 shown in same patient, on right.

Trauma

- CT scan is best for revealing unsuspected vertical vertebral body fractures and neural arch fractures. Oblique CT reconstruction of cervical spine shows facet joint dislocations with greater clarity.
- MRI shows changes in spinal cord which suggest physiological transection (high signal in T2). **Also, high signal in T2 in all soft tissues on sagittal views would suggest a major antero-posterior soft tissue disruption and associated long term danger to the cord.**
- There is a current vogue for classifications of devilish and pointless complexity, based on a combination of severity of bone and soft tissue damage, and enormous presumption as to mode of injury [3,4]. THESE CLASSIFICATIONS ARE THEN USED TO JUSTIFY COMPLEX SURGICAL PROCEDURES USUALLY INVOLVING EXPENSIVE IMPLANTS, AND OFTEN IN THE MISTAKEN ASSUMPTION THAT SURGERY ALONE CAN IMPROVE NEUROLOGICAL DEFICIT. THERE IS A WIDESPREAD UNFORTUNATE AMNESIA FOR THE OLDER (BÖHLER) EVIDENCE THAT SPONTANEOUS HEALING CAN ACHIEVE MUCH WITHOUT SURGERY [5-10].
- Of greater importance is the ability to record a meticulous neurological examination, irrespective of the classification in fashion.
- **The imaging investigations show us only the last frame of a movie we never saw.**

Management Acute/Early (assuming all other injuries stable and patient conscious)
- Without paralysis: <u>pain</u> control; <u>bracing</u> for safety of cord (seldom required except for neck injuries); <u>mobilise</u> as soon as pain allows; <u>reduce</u> cervical dislocation by graduated increase in skull traction, provided injury no more than 48 hours old. Thereafter, leave dislocated, or reduce surgically and fix/fuse.
- With paralysis: urinary catheter; respiration adequate (oxygen saturation) in high paralysis; pain control; posture to minimise skin pressure, and frequent change using many trained hands; antacid equivalents to prevent gastric stress ulceration; monitor blood pressure frequently; immobilise as necessary to protect cord from further damage, including skull traction when necessary; monitor neurological status daily/twice daily and chart; prevent constipation with aperients and/or suppositories.

High dose corticosteroids now considered unhelpful and positively dangerous [11,12]. **Surgery indicated** at this stage only if: - there is progressive loss of neurology (decompression and fusion, preferably by anterior approach, at whatever level in the spine).
    - there is a sufficient disruption of the spinal column to render any safe mobilisation impossible (anterior or posterior approach to fix and fuse).

Management Post-acute/Late
- Without paralysis: Plain flexion/extension lateral x-rays 6-8 weeks later, under patient's control. If excessive subluxation or horizontal translation still present (cervical spine); or progressive kyphosis (thoracic and lumbar spine) = indication for fusion surgery to prevent even further deformity especially in presence of persistent pain.

    Massive posterior shunt of bone into spinal canal <u>will</u> spontaneously remodel to clear canal within approximately 24 months [8,10].

    Continue to mobilise to full fitness.
    Late indications for fusion surgery = one or more of: intractable pain, progressive deformity, increasing neurological deficit **("PPP" = Pain, Posture, Paralysis).**

- With paralysis: Watch for spasticity = end of "spinal shock". Involuntary persistent spasms very distressing: manage with oral medication and possibly injected botulinum toxin or intrathecal baclofen. Wheelchair specification and training. Likewise intermittent self catheterisation; skin care; urine testing for infection. Increased spasticity and sweats suggest infection somewhere. Gastric mucosal protection against stress ulceration.
    Late indications for fusion surgery = one or more of: intractable pain, progressive deformity, increasing neurological deficit **("PPP" = Pain, Posture, Paralysis).**

    Lifelong regular follow-up is the ideal.

Trauma

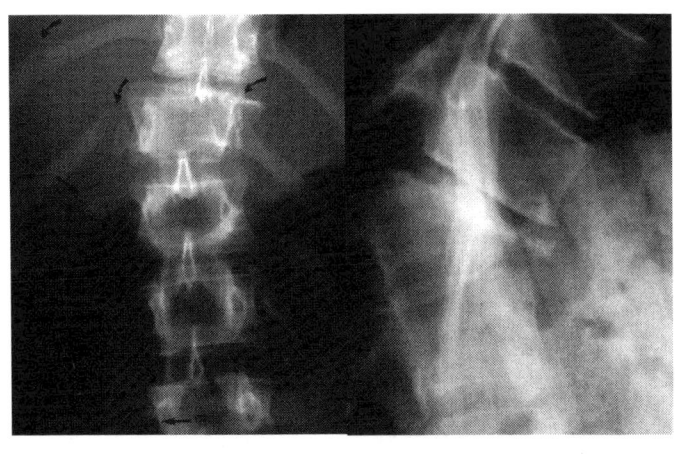

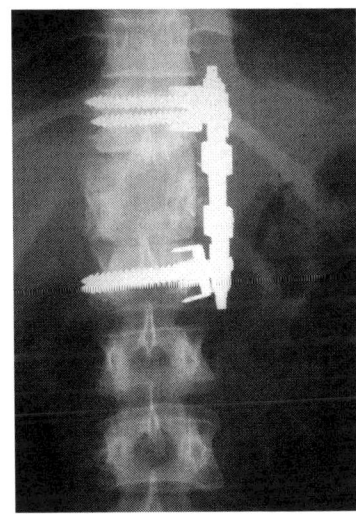 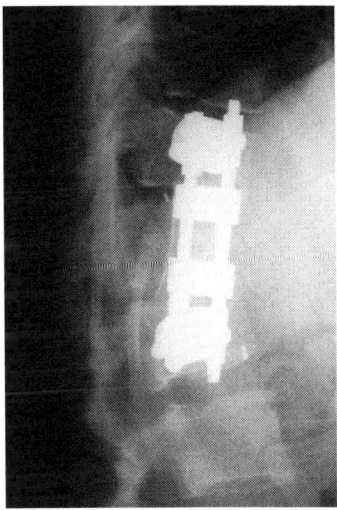

Frankel A paralysis after poor handling at roadside following RTA.
Top left: fractured rib and lateral subluxation T11/12 - severe injury.
Top right: T12 wedge deformity, 45° painful gibbus.
Bottom left: Kaneda fixation T11-L1 anterior. Tricortical iliac crest graft.
Bottom right: Gibbus corrected to 15°; pain free, but paralysis permanent.

Complications of spinal cord injury with paralysis:-
- Urinary tract infection: repeated infection with nephritis and renal failure = most likely but preventable cause of early death.
- Pressure sores with infection.
- Spasms in lower limbs.
- Deformity: kyphosis and/or scoliosis at fracture site; long curve of paralytic scoliosis.·
- Pain: at fracture site; with or without syringomyelia.
- Syringomyelia: cystic degeneration of spinal cord at site of injury, with burning local pain, loss of dermatomes, sweating.

Prognosis
Wide range of possibility of return of useful walking ability, 5% to 80% of patients, depending on the density and segmental level of the injury, as well as on the quality of management.

References:

1. *El Masry WS. Physiologic instability of the spinal cord following injury. Paraplegia 31:273-27, 1993.*
2. *Frankel HL, Hancock D, Hyslop G et al. The value of postural reduction in the initial management of closed injuries of the spine with paraplegia and tetraplegia. 1. Paraplegia 7 :179-92, 1969.*
3. *Magerl F, Aebi M, Gertzbein S et al. A comprehensive classification of thoracic and lumbar injuries. Eur Spine J 3:184-201, 1994.*
4. *Vaccaro A, Lehman R, Hurlbert R et al. A new classification of thoracolumbar injuries: the importance of injury morphology, the integrity of the posterior ligamentous complex, and neurologic status. Spine 30:2325-33, 2005.*
5. *Lorenz Böhler film 1933; naked men in plaster jackets performing amazing feats of brute strength after severe spinal injuries treated without surgery.*

6. Katoh S et al. The neurologic outcome in conservatively treated patients with incomplete closed traumatic cervical spinal cord injuries. Spine. 21:2345-2351, 1996.
7. Jaffray DC. Why operate on a spinal fracture? Watson-Jones Lecture. British Orthopaedic Association annual meeting, Manchester 2004. Thirty patients with spinal injuries definable as "unstable" by any scheme or classification, without neurological deficit, mobilised without surgery within 3 to 6 months, to "running, jumping, and standing still".
8. Wood K, Buttermann G, Mehbod A et al. Operative compared with nonoperative treatment of a thoracolumbar burst fracture without neurological deficit. A prospective, randomised study. J Bone Joint Surg Am. 85-A:773-81, 2003.
9. Chow G, Nelson B, Gebhard J et al. Functional outcome of thoracolumbar burst fractures managed with hyperextension casting or bracing and early mobilization. Spine. 21:2170-05, 1996.
10. Mumford J, Weinstein J et al. Thoracolumbar burst fractures. The clinical efficacy and outcome of nonoperative management. Spine. 18:955-70, 1993.
11. Short D, El Masry W, Jones P. High dose methylprednisolone in the management of acute spinal cord injury – a systematic review from a clinical perspective. Spinal Cord 38:273-86, 2000.
12. Qian T, Guo X, Levi AD et al. High-dose methylprednisolone may cause myopathy in acute spinal cord injury patients. Spinal Cord 43:199-203, 2005.

TUMOUR – PRIMARY

1. Primary tumours of the spine are uncommon (1:5) in comparison with secondary (metastatic) tumours spread from breast, prostate, lung, kidney, thyroid, adenomas of unknown origin.

2. Tissues of origin reflect the diversity of primary spine tumours: bone (including marrow), cartilage, connective, neural.

3. Malignant more common than benign.

4. **Most common is myeloma**, cancer of plasma cells of haemopoietic bone marrow.
   - Proliferation of plasma ("cartwheel") cells in bone marrow.
   - "Multiple myeloma", if found in several sites in thoracic spine, in patients over 50, commonly including skull with typical punched-out lytic defects.
   - "Plasmacytoma", if found in a single vertebral body, as a typical uniformly flattened "pancake" vertebra.
   - Clinical presentation = pain, kyphosis deformity, neurological deficit.
   - Investigations (in Multiple): Anaemia; ESR > 100; Bence-Jones proteinuria; raised IgG; raised serum calcium; bone marrow histology. Isotope scan typically negative. Bone marrow aspiration and bone biopsy.
   - Treatment: Plasmacytoma = radiotherapy and chemotherapy: good prognosis.
   - Multiple myeloma = radiotherapy and chemotherapy: poor prognosis. Surgical decompression of cord and nerve roots may be possible, combined with some stabilization.

5. Other malignant tumours:
   - Osteosarcoma (from osteoblasts; teenagers; pain and neurological deficit; lysis and sclerosis; biopsy; surgery and chemotherapy; lung metastases, lethal).
   - Chondrosarcoma (from chondrocytes; middle age; lumbosacral; mimics disc prolapse; large lytic zones with spotty calcification; biopsy; aggressive surgery; <50% 5 year survival).

Tumour – Primary

- Glioma (astrocytoma, glioblastoma, oligodendroglioma); rare, brain more than spine.
- Chordoma (from sacrococcygeal notochordal remnants; pelvic mass; sacrococcygeal pain and rectal dysfunction; wide local destruction; may metastasise; surgical excision if possible but recurrence typical).
- Schwannoma, neurofibroma (from Schwann cells; cauda equina; intradural on posterior nerve root; back pain and sciatica; surgical excision).
- Ewing's tumour (young men; pain and neurological deficit; necrotic foci; combine surgery, radiation, chemotherapy; lung metastases, lethal).
- Ependymoma (from cells lining cord central canal, cauda equina and filum terminale; back pain and sciatica; pre-sacral mass; surgical excision).

6. Benign tumours are:
   - Haemangioma (most common, present in 11% of autopsy spines, spherical T2 defects in vertebral bodies, usually symptomless);
   - Osteoid osteoma (posterior arch, painful scoliosis);
   - Osteoblastoma (posterior arch, painful scoliosis);
   - Giant cell tumour (sacrum, extensive local destruction).
   - Aneurysmal bone cyst (lumbar neural arch, massive cystic destruction).
   - Neurofibroma.

TUMOUR - METASTASIS
[G. a removing; remote from]

1. Spread of primary (cancer of origin) to bone at sites remote from primary.
2. Metastasis to bone indicates **stage** 4/4 of development of cancer.
3. Spread is probably haematogenous eg prostate carcinoma to spine via **Batson**'s venous plexus.
4. Commonest primaries metastasising to spine: breast, prostate, lung, kidney, thyroid, "adenocarcinoma of unknown origin".
5. Commonest site in spine is thoracolumbar junction vertebrae.
6. Survival related more to nature and histology (**grade**) of primary rather than staging. "Breast is best". Lung (bronchogenic) is worst.

Presentation
- PPP = **P**ain in spine; **P**ostural deformity eg Kyphosis; **P**aralysis of varying degree, in lower limbs and sphincters.
- RED FLAGS: known primary cancer, constant pain, worse at night, middle age onwards, loss of appetite and weight, sudden recent deformity, lower limb weakness and **paraesthesiae,** loss of perineal sphincter function.
- Any age group, but childhood cancers are relatively rare in spine.
- Gender largely dependent on diagnosis: breast and prostate primaries are two of the commonest.
- Differential diagnosis on presentation: major disc prolapse with cauda equina compression; spinal stenosis; infective discitis with adjacent osteitis; osteoporosis with wedge compression fracture of vertebrae.

Tumour Metastasis

Diagnosis
- Plain x-rays may show vertebral deformity on lateral; on anterior view "winking owl or blind owl" of pedicle destruction ; lung metastasis in chest x-ray.

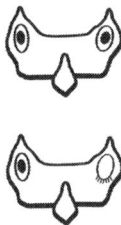

- Plain x-rays show disc height remarkably well preserved even when adjacent vertebrae show major destruction.

    Distinct from **infection** where disc equally damaged. Aphorism: "Good disc, bad news. Bad disc, good news" insofar as infection may be regarded as preferable to cancer.
- Radio-isotope bone scan (Technetium^{99m}; whole body) to show extent of skeletal mets: "black measles" describes widespread mets and poor prognosis.

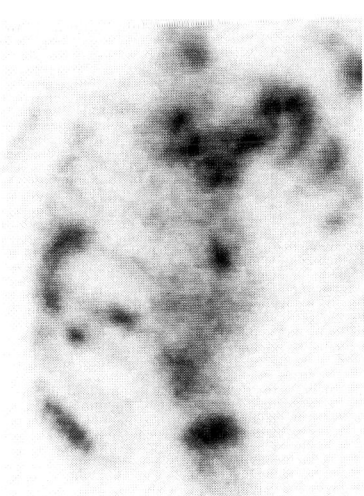

Radioisotope scan of chest AP middle-aged man with mulitple metastases to ribs and sternum from prostrate.

- MRI whole spine: infiltrative changes in vertebrae, even those vertebrae not deformed on plain x-ray; extrusion of tumour mass into spinal canal and degree of threat to cord or cauda equina. Axial views may show kidney primary. Disc preservation shown on plain x-ray, confirmed on MRI.
- CT scan of chest to exclude primary and lung metastases.
- CT scan or Ultrasound of abdomen to exclude visceral metastases, especially liver.
- Biopsy by CT-guided needle of affected vertebra.
- Bone marrow biopsy if myeloma or lymphoma suspected.
- Check serum for immunoglobulins (electrophoresis) to exclude myelomas.

Treatment
- Requires whole oncology team to assess worth of various combinations of chemotherapy and radiotherapy customised for particular cancer diagnosed.
- Radiotherapy and bisphosphonates frequently best for urgent control of refractory pain.
- Check serum for hypercalcaemia and correct as necessary.
- Surgical excision of infiltrated vertebra and stabilisation, provided that: Patient in good general condition. Isolated metastasis. No discoverable visceral metastases. Not primary lung, stomach or bladder cancer (very poor prognosis). Threat to neurology (on MRI).
  No major paralysis (very seldom reversible by surgery); and continent.
- Above conditions embody Tokuhashi principles of prognosis (1990). Items score 2 (good); 0 (bad); and 1 for somewhere in between. Total score of 9-12 justifies major surgical effort; less than 5 justifies palliation only; uncertain prognosis 5-9 (Page 188).
- Purpose of surgery: to provide best possible quality of life for time remaining and preserve continence. Expect minimum 3 months' survival to allow for postoperative recovery and return home. Death in hospital is a kind of failure of management.
- Preoperative embolisation of tumour feeder vessels for very vascular renal metastases.

Tumour Metastasis

Techniques of surgery
- Anterior approach for mainly anterior destruction: transthoracic, transdiaphragmatic, intra-abdominal, as required.
- Posterior approach for mainly posterior destruction. Excise as much vertebra/tumour as will leave spinal cord free.
- Anterior: Stabilise with some bone or artificial strut bridging into healthy vertebrae plus screw/plate fixation.
- Posterior: Stabilise with rod/screw/hook/frame and-wire fixation bridging across surgical defect. Combined anterior and posterior: for extra stability.

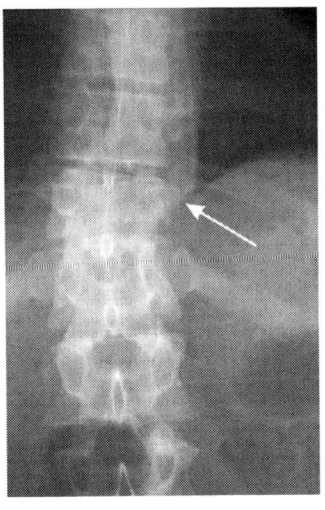 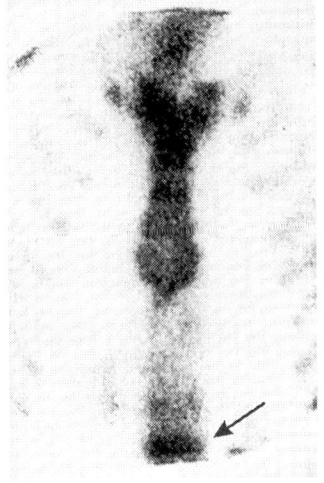

Partial collapse T11 with loss of left pedicle (arrowed) = "winking owl" sign.

Radio-isotope scan shows increased uptake at T11 (arrowed).

Tumour Metastasis

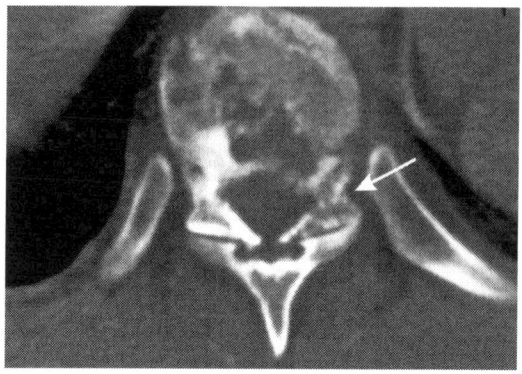

Destruction of part of vertbral body T11 and left pedicle (arrowed). CT scan good for bone detail.

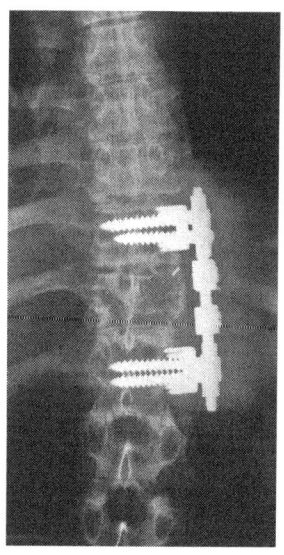

Double rod and screw fixation T10-T12 over a tricortical strut, left.

TOKUHASHI SCORE FOR PROGNOSIS IN SPINE METASTATIC DISEASE

Item	Description	Score
1	General Condition (Karnofsky 1967)*	
	Poor	0
	Moderate	1
	Good	2
2	Extraspinal Mets	
	3+	0
	1-2	1
	0	2
3	Vertebral Body Mets	
	3+	0
	2	1
	1	2
4	Visceral Mets	
	Non-resectable	0
	Resectable	1
	No Mets	2
5	Primary	
	Lung, Stomach	0
	Kidney, Liver, Uterus, Unknown	1
	Thyroid, Prostate, Breast, Rectum	2
6	Spinal Cord Paralysis	
	Complete	0
	Incomplete	1
	No Neuro Deficit	2
	Best Prognosis Score =	12

Interpretation:
Scores 0-5 = survival beyond 3 months unlikely: palliative surgery only (if any).
Scores 5-9 = survival 3-12 months: grey zone: palliative or excisional surgery.
Scores 9-12 = survival 12 + months: excisional surgery.

Reference:
Tokuhashi Y, Matsuzaki H, Toriyama S, Kawano H, Ohsaka S. Scoring system for the preoperative evaluation of metastatic spine tumour prognosis. Spine 15:1110-13, 1990.

Karnofsky DA. Clinical evaluation of anticancer drugs. Cancer chemotherapy. GANN Monograph 2:223-31, 1967.
A Performance Scale Index crudely divided into 3 categories: equivalent to institutionalised and unable to care for self; unable to work but personal care possible; normal work and personal care activities.

Oxford Textbook of Palliative Medicine, Oxford University Press, 1993; 109.

www.hospicepatients.org/karnofsky.html

WHIPLASH

- Describes both the forces as well as the consequences of a specific type of soft tissue injury to the cervical spine. The term applies almost always to the result of a rear-end shunt road accident. Because the head weighs 4.5 to 5 kgs (10 lbs), balanced somewhat precariously at the top of the slender cervical spine, any sudden displacing force could impose severe strain on the soft tissue stabilisers (muscles and ligaments) of the cervical spine, as well as a sprain of intervertebral facet joints.

- "Whiplash" is intended to describe the anteroposterior movements of the head during the shunt, and then the painful long term disability which sometimes follows. The term is over-dramatic; an ankle sprain may have more severe consequences but is almost never attributable to a compensable misdemeanour committed by another. "Whiplash" is likely to elicit greater sympathy in court or in legal correspondence, than mere "neck strain/sprain". Attempts to abolish use of the term are bound to fail.

- By definition, whiplash excludes identifiable and specific fresh injury of a kind which could be diagnosed on x-ray, or suggested by finding fresh neurological deficit. The subject is therefore fraught with difficulty, not because of the medical consequences but because of the medicolegal and financial consequences. The disability associated with the injury is said to vary considerably from one national culture to another. The degree of disability can be judged only on the word of the victim.

- The vast majority of patients will complain of neck pain and stiffness sufficient to prevent safe driving, sleep, and physical work for weeks to months after injury. There may be some pain radiation to shoulders and upper limbs. Any suggestion of an upper motor neurone syndrome or a cervical radiculopathy, would require further investigation by MRI or intrathecal contrast. In the event of finding cord or cervical root compression, or fracture/dislocation, the condition then disqualifies itself from "whiplash".

- In general, the symptoms dissipate gradually over two years. It is not possible to be dogmatic as to the long term consequences of this injury: advanced spondylosis is so common in the middle aged and elderly population, that it would not be possible to ascribe later spondylosis to the injury, with any certainty. Analgesics, cervical spine support of short duration (weeks rather than months), and physiotherapy should see most patients through to near full recovery within two years.

WOUND INFECTION

[see also COMPLICATIONS]

- Most likely originates elsewhere within the patient from some cryptic asymptomatic source (ear? tooth?) but increasingly contamination from ward or theatre environment.
Organism most likely = Staphylococcus aureus, especially methicillin resistant variety (MRSA). Said to be more common in general hospitals than in elective specialty hospitals. Clostridium difficile less common but carries a high mortality rate. Protracted periods of tissue retraction may predispose to infection. **Diabetes is associated with highest independent risk of surgical site infection** *(Olsen MA, Nepple JJ, Riew KD et al. J Bone Joint Surg Am 2008, 90:62-9).*

- Prophylaxis in practice consists of frequent alcohol handwash by all hospital staff in all clinical areas; laminar flow ventilation in theatre; pre-operative broad spectrum antibiotics; antibiotic wound washout at frequent intervals during surgery. Effectiveness of these measures probably not quantified.

- Treatment requires identification of infecting organism; meticulous surgical debridement of infected and necrotic tissue including obviously necrotic bone and bone graft; application of antibiotics based on organism sensitivity, in large doses of those likely to cope with MRSA (vancomycin and linezolid presently). Metronidazole and vancomycin for C diff. **PICC** line = best means of delivery. Vital internal fixation should be left in situ at this stage.

- Difficult decision then as to whether to leave wound open, packed with swabs soaked in antiseptic medium and allow to granulate till ready for secondary suture, or whether to close over some antibiotic irrigation system. Guide: close wound if relatively superficial. If infection down to bone, best to leave to granulate and repeat debridement as often as necessary.

- **Vacuum pump very useful if open wound slow to granulate.**

X-RAYS

(See IMAGING)

ZOSTER
[G. zoster = girdle]

Herpes Zoster ("shingles") is an extremely painful condition in the dermatome of an affected nerve root. It is the result of reactivation of a previous chicken pox virus infection, varicella zoster, from within a nerve root ganglion. After the start of the root pain there is a vesicular (blistering) eruption in the skin of the dermatome, and redness. Intercostal nerves are most commonly affected, but involvement of lumbar and sacral roots is possible and may present as a puzzling cause of sciatica. Reactivation may be spontaneous in the middle-aged and elderly, but may be due to immunosuppression as in malignancy and AIDS.

Treatment with oral acyclovir is useful if started early.
Give systemically for the immunocompromised.
Post-herpetic neuralgia is almost refractory to treatment.

Printed in Great Britain
by Amazon